Barbara Bernard

Routine Kills

The arrival of indifference in the
modern healthcare system

bup

Barbara Bernard

Routine Kills

The arrival of indifference in the modern healthcare system

ISBN: 978-3-69035-632-9 (Paperback)
ISBN: 978-3-69035-637-4 (e-book)
Order number: 2013.2

Cover design: Kerstin Laube

Bremen University Press, 2025.
Fahrenheitstr. 11
28359 Bremen
bup@bremenuniversitypress.com
www.bremenuniversitypress.com

The manuscript may not be used in whole or in part without the prior written consent of the publisher.

This book was printed on environmentally friendly paper from sustainable forestry in order to conserve resources and minimise environmental impact. By using recycled materials and FSC-certified paper, we are helping to protect forests and reduce our ecological footprint.

Barbara Bernard

Routine Kills

The arrival of indifference in the
modern healthcare system

Overview

FOREWORD	14
CHAPTER 1: MODERN MEDICINE BETWEEN PROGRESS AND ALIENATION	15
CHAPTER 2: WHAT IS INDIFFERENCE? A PSYCHOLOGICAL AND ETHICAL APPROACH	19
CHAPTER 3: WHEN ROUTINE BECOMES A TRAP - MECHANISMS OF BLUNTING	26
CHAPTER 4: STRUCTURAL CAUSES OF MEDICAL INDIFFERENCE	33
CHAPTER 5: THE INVISIBLE VICTIMS - WHEN THE PERSON BEHIND THE CASE DISAPPEARS	40
CHAPTER 6: SILENT BRUTALISATION - INDIFFERENCE AS A SOCIAL PHENOMENON IN A TEAM	47
CHAPTER 7: TRAINING WITHOUT ATTITUDE? THE ROLE OF MEDICAL TEACHING	54
CHAPTER 8: INDIFFERENCE AS A PROTECTIVE MECHANISM - NECESSARY OR DANGEROUS?	61
CHAPTER 9: WHEN SYSTEMS BECOME BLUNT - INSTITUTIONAL INDIFFERENCE AS AN EXPRESSION OF STRUCTURAL FAILURE	67
CHAPTER 10: SUFFERING WITHOUT ECHO - THE PATIENTS' PERSPECTIVE	74

CHAPTER 11: WHEN CARERS FALL SILENT - THE SILENT EXHAUSTION OF THE HELPING PROFESSIONS 80

CHAPTER 12: THE DANGEROUS POWER OF HABITUATION - HOW NORMALITY BREEDS INDIFFERENCE 86

CHAPTER 13: THE ROLE OF LANGUAGE - WHEN WORDS DEHUMANISE 92

CHAPTER 14: LACK OF ETHICS AS A SYSTEM ERROR - WHEN MORAL ORIENTATION IS LOST 98

CHAPTER 15: WHEN THE SYSTEM MAKES YOU ILL - BURNOUT, DEPRESSION AND MORAL EXHAUSTION IN THE HEALTHCARE SYSTEM 104

CHAPTER 16: THE GREAT SILENCE - WHY INDIFFERENCE IS NOT TALKED ABOUT 113

CHAPTER 17: SILENT CONNIVANCE - HOW INDIFFERENCE BECOMES ENTRENCHED IN TEAMS 119

CHAPTER 18: THE RETURN OF COMPASSION - WHAT HELPS AGAINST INDIFFERENCE 125

CHAPTER 19: BETWEEN ASPIRATION AND REALITY - WHY HUMANITY IS NOT A SURE-FIRE SUCCESS 131

CHAPTER 20: WHAT REMAINS - THE DECISION FOR HUMANITY AS DAILY PRACTICE 139

PRESERVING HUMANITY - DESPITE EVERYTHING 144

OUTLOOK: A MEDICINE THAT HEALS - NOT JUST THE BODY 146

6

Table of contents

FOREWORD	**14**
CHAPTER 1: MODERN MEDICINE BETWEEN PROGRESS AND ALIENATION	**15**
CHAPTER 2: WHAT IS INDIFFERENCE? A PSYCHOLOGICAL AND ETHICAL APPROACH	**19**
1. Definition: Indifference as an emotional, moral and social state	19
2. Differentiation from related phenomena: Lack of empathy, burnout, cynicism	20
3. Indifference as a moral failure or functional strategy?	22
4. The ethical relevance of emotional apathy in the medical profession	23
5. Philosophical concepts of indifference and their significance for medicine	24
CHAPTER 3: WHEN ROUTINE BECOMES A TRAP - MECHANISMS OF BLUNTING	**26**
1. Everyday life in the clinic and practice: routines as structure and stress	26
2. Cognitive and emotional effects of monotonous sequences of actions	27
3. Automation of medical decisions and loss of compassion	29
4. The role of time pressure, shift systems and economic targets	30
5. How a sense of responsibility dissolves under routine conditions	31

CHAPTER 4: STRUCTURAL CAUSES OF MEDICAL INDIFFERENCE 33

1. Healthcare systems under the primacy of economics 33
2. Staff shortages and excessive demands are the norm 34
3. Bureaucracy, documentation requirements and digital interfaces 35
4. False incentives in the remuneration of medical services 37
5. Organisational coldness: Hospitals as companies instead of places of healing 38

CHAPTER 5: THE INVISIBLE VICTIMS - WHEN THE PERSON BEHIND THE CASE DISAPPEARS 40

1. The view through the case number: depersonalisation in patient care 40
2. Subtle violence through ignorance, lack of time and disregard 41
3. Psychological stress due to symptoms that are not taken seriously 42
4. The fatal dynamic between medical indifference and patient mistrust 44
5. Reports from the field: voices of patients and relatives 45

CHAPTER 6: SILENT BRUTALISATION - INDIFFERENCE AS A SOCIAL PHENOMENON IN A TEAM 47

1. Group dynamics in medical hierarchies 47
2. Cynicism as a collective protective wall against emotional overload 48
3. Silence, complicity and the disappearance of moral responsibility 49
4. Social sanctions against empathetic colleagues 51

5.	A culture of looking the other way: when misbehaviour becomes the norm	52

CHAPTER 7: TRAINING WITHOUT ATTITUDE? THE ROLE OF MEDICAL TEACHING — 54

1.	Academisation versus humanity: curricula without empathy training	54
2.	Examination culture, grade pressure and the decoupling of theory and practice	55
3.	Early indoctrination into a system of efficiency and objectivity	57
4.	Empathy as a "soft skill" or an indispensable competence?	58
5.	Approaches for an ethical-emotional educational reform in medical training	59

CHAPTER 8: INDIFFERENCE AS A PROTECTIVE MECHANISM - NECESSARY OR DANGEROUS? — 61

1.	Psychological protection strategies in high-stress professions	61
2.	The boundary between self-protection and emotional coldness	62
3.	Empathy as a risk: emotional exhaustion through closeness	63
4.	The role of promoting resilience in professional self-care	64
5.	Possibilities of demarcation without ethical withdrawal	65

CHAPTER 9: WHEN SYSTEMS BECOME BLUNT - INSTITUTIONAL INDIFFERENCE AS AN EXPRESSION OF STRUCTURAL FAILURE — 67

1.	From attitude to structure: How organisations create indifference	67
2.	The logic of the system: efficiency, control, standardisation	68
3.	The role of leadership and management culture	69

4.	Organisational blindness for the subjective	71
5.	Ways out of structural blunting	72

CHAPTER 10: SUFFERING WITHOUT ECHO - THE PATIENTS' PERSPECTIVE — 74

1.	The experience of being unseen during the course of the disease	74
2.	Speechlessness, isolation and the loss of subjectivity	75
3.	Violations through silence, avoidance and functional communication	76
4.	The search for meaning, comfort and support in the medical system	77
5.	The desire for encounters and the longing for dignity	78

CHAPTER 11: WHEN CARERS FALL SILENT - THE SILENT EXHAUSTION OF THE HELPING PROFESSIONS — 80

1.	Proximity to suffering as a daily challenge	80
2.	The moral stress between knowing, wanting and not being able to	81
3.	Devaluation, hierarchy and the invisibility of nursing expertise	82
4.	The retreat into the functional role as a survival strategy	83
5.	The silent cry for help: Why indifference is also a sign of pain	85

CHAPTER 12: THE DANGEROUS POWER OF HABITUATION - HOW NORMALITY BREEDS INDIFFERENCE — 86

1.	The process of blunting through repetition	86
2.	When the extraordinary becomes commonplace	87
3.	The creeping shift in moral standards	88
4.	The social protection of the "insensitive"	89

5.	Ways back to ethical vigilance in everyday life	90

CHAPTER 13: THE ROLE OF LANGUAGE - WHEN WORDS DEHUMANISE — 92

1.	Language as a mirror of inner attitude	92
2.	The loss of personal contact in everyday clinical practice	93
3.	Euphemisms, abbreviations and the loss of depth	94
4.	Linguistic distance as a form of professional self-relief	95
5.	Ways to a more human language in the medical context	96

CHAPTER 14: LACK OF ETHICS AS A SYSTEM ERROR - WHEN MORAL ORIENTATION IS LOST — 98

1.	Medicine as an ethically charged practice	98
2.	The invisibility of ethical issues in everyday clinical practice	99
3.	Economisation, hierarchy and ethical speechlessness	100
4.	Ethics as individual responsibility or collective practice?	101
5.	Steps towards the ethical re-centring of medical practice	102

CHAPTER 15: WHEN THE SYSTEM MAKES YOU ILL - BURNOUT, DEPRESSION AND MORAL EXHAUSTION IN THE HEALTHCARE SYSTEM — 104

1.	The healthcare system as a high-risk environment for mental exhaustion	104
2.	Burnout as a collapse between commitment and reality	105
3.	Moral exhaustion - when acting against your own convictions makes you ill	106
4.	Depression as an expression of silent despair in the system	107
5.	From symptom to change - an appeal to the system	108
6.	Structural prevention - how systems can remain human	109

CHAPTER 16: THE GREAT SILENCE - WHY INDIFFERENCE IS NOT TALKED ABOUT — 113

1. Indifference as a blind spot of the institution — 113
2. Fear of your own sensitivity — 114
3. The normalisation of the deviant — 115
5. Ways out of silence - The return to language — 117

CHAPTER 17: SILENT CONNIVANCE - HOW INDIFFERENCE BECOMES ENTRENCHED IN TEAMS — 119

1. The individual in the collective - How moral impulses get lost — 119
2. Group norms and the principle of unspoken consensus — 120
3. Loyalty as a moral dilemma — 121
4. The dynamics of collective displacement — 122
5. Ways out of the silent complicity — 123

CHAPTER 18: THE RETURN OF COMPASSION - WHAT HELPS AGAINST INDIFFERENCE — 125

1. Compassion as a reconstructive force in the face of the systemic — 125
2. The neurobiology of resonance - compassion as a natural disposition — 126
3. The ethics of small steps - compassion as a means of action — 127
4. Collective empathy - when systems become healing — 128
5. Reconnecting with the origin — 129

CHAPTER 19: BETWEEN ASPIRATION AND REALITY - WHY HUMANITY IS NOT A SURE-FIRE SUCCESS — 131

1. The myth of the good - between vocation and excessive demands — 131

2.	The institutional staging of humanity - façade or substance?	132
3.	The psychodynamic price of the functional self	133
4.	The ethical erosion caused by structural violence	134
5.	The path to authenticity - between self-knowledge and structural criticism	135
6.	Maturing humanity - a path through ambivalence	136

CHAPTER 20: WHAT REMAINS - THE DECISION FOR HUMANITY AS DAILY PRACTICE — **139**

1.	The decision as a daily act of resistance	139
2.	The unfinished ethics - humanity as an imposition	140
3.	Self-care as a prerequisite for ethical presence	141
4.	The silent responsibility of the institution	142
5.	What remains - in the depths	143

PRESERVING HUMANITY - DESPITE EVERYTHING — **144**

OUTLOOK: A MEDICINE THAT HEALS - NOT JUST THE BODY — **146**

Foreword

It often begins quietly. A look that is no longer searching. A question that is no longer asked. A symptom that is forced into prefabricated templates. In modern medicine, repetition is commonplace, procedures are optimised, processes standardised. But with routine, a dangerous companion creeps in: indifference. Not out of malice, but out of exhaustion, time pressure and a culture that prioritises efficiency over empathy. Where once there was curiosity and care, a clinical vacuum is created - sterile, correct, but empty.

This book invites us to pause for thought. It asks uncomfortable questions where habits have taken on a life of their own. It looks for the fine cracks in the system where humanity is lost - not through failure, but through too much routine. Because where the special is overlooked in the everyday, where the person disappears behind the diagnosis, a situation arises that can jeopardise lives.

This study is not an attack, but a call. A call to return to what medicine should be at its core: a human art borne by responsibility, attentiveness and the ability to see the new even in the familiar.

Chapter 1: Modern medicine between progress and alienation

The history of medicine is closely linked to the human quest for knowledge, healing and overcoming suffering. Since the beginnings of the art of healing, medical practice has not only been characterised by technical knowledge, but also by the ethical ideal of care and attention. The physician was not only regarded as a user of medical procedures, but above all as a companion in suffering, as an interpreter of the experience of illness and as a moral agent in the service of the sick person. With the advent of modern technologies, the increasing rationalisation of medical procedures and the economic penetration of the healthcare system, this image has changed fundamentally. Today, modern medicine is caught between progressive efficiency and growing alienation, between precise diagnostics and the loss of personal closeness, between standardised high-performance care and the disappearance of the human being as a subject.

The progress of medicine in the twentieth and twenty-first centuries has been remarkable in many respects. Diseases that were once considered incurable can now be controlled or cured. Surgical techniques have become more precise, diagnoses more reliable thanks to imaging techniques, and molecular medicine provides insights into disease mechanisms that would have been unthinkable just a few decades ago. These developments are an expression of a scientific and technological success that has prolonged the lives of many people and improved their quality of life. At the same time, however, a new form of distance has crept in with this progress, which is not technical but anthropological in nature. The question of the person behind the data, the subjectivity of illness and the dialogue dimension of healing has increasingly been pushed into the background.

The mechanisation of medicine is accompanied by a depersonalisation that manifests itself not only in clinical practice, but also in the language and thinking of doctors. Patients become cases, organs become targets of therapeutic interventions, diagnoses become algorithmic decision nodes. The doctor-patient relationship is increasingly interrupted by the dominance of technical interfaces. Where previously the focus was on the consultation, the physical examination and the observation of the whole person, today laboratory values, image data and digitalised anamnesis masks determine everyday clinical practice. As a result of these changes, what could be described as the human dimension of medical practice is disappearing - that fragile but fundamental connection between two people, one of whom is ill and the other of whom is healing.

Another aspect of alienation lies in the increasing standardisation of medical procedures. Quality management, evidence-based guidelines and checklists may seem sensible from a health economics and safety perspective, but they also carry the risk of marginalising individual characteristics and subjective experiences of illness. The patient is no longer considered as a whole, but categorised and treated according to fixed parameters. This rationalisation, as helpful as it may be in avoiding errors, runs the risk of blotting out the personal, the situational and the dialogically unpredictable aspects of the medical process. What does not fit into the grid is overlooked or perceived as disruptive.

In addition, the economisation of the healthcare system has significantly increased the pressure on medical staff. Hospitals have to work economically, doctors are subject to production figures and nursing staff are controlled by clocking and cost efficiency. These structural conditions contribute significantly to the fact that time has become a scarce commodity. The encounter with the patient, the conversation, the listening - everything that gives meaning to suffering and enables trust - is increasingly displaced by administrative duties and time pressure. The alienation of medicine is therefore not just a cultural or individual phenomenon, but an expression of a comprehensive system change in which economic logic increasingly determines the patterns of action in healthcare.

In the midst of these developments, the question arises as to what has become of the original self-image of healing. Can a medicine that defines itself primarily in terms of efficiency, technology and organisation still do justice to the claim of doing justice to the suffering person? Or does this progress in its current form lead to a creeping indifference because the personal dimension of healing is lost from view? Modern medicine is at a crossroads: either it succeeds in combining the achievements of progress with a new form of care and empathy - or it runs the risk of losing its ethical substance and therefore its credibility.

This book explores the question of how indifference can become established in a system that is originally committed to life. It examines how structures, routines and ways of thinking can lead to attention, mindfulness and compassion being systematically suppressed or ignored. In this field of tension between technological excellence and human numbness, the analysis begins with a close look at the psychological and ethical foundations of the term "indifference".

Chapter 2: What is indifference? A psychological and ethical approach

1. Definition: indifference as an emotional, moral and social state

The term indifference has negative connotations in everyday language and is often associated with emotional coldness, lack of interest or withdrawal. However, a precise conceptualisation shows that it is a multi-layered phenomenon that can be described on several levels. Indifference can be understood as an emotional reaction - or more precisely: the absence of such a reaction - in which external stimuli that would normally trigger compassion or engagement no longer evoke an inner response. It thus describes a kind of emotional blunting in which those affected no longer react sensitively to suffering, danger or injustice.

At the same time, indifference can also be understood as a moral state. It refers to a suspension of ethical attention, a lack of a sense of responsibility and a failure to turn to the other as a subject. Those who act indifferently decide - whether consciously or unconsciously - not to take an interest in the well-being of others and evade the moral duty to sympathise. In this respect, indifference has a deep ethical structure: it is not merely the absence of emotion, but the expression of a certain attitude towards the world and fellow human beings.

After all, indifference is also a social phenomenon. In interpersonal contexts, it has an excluding and degrading effect. Anyone who treats another person with indifference implicitly denies them social recognition. Indifference is hurtful because it marks the other person as meaningless. In social systems such as medicine, where recognition and attention are constitutive for the success of the relationship, indifference therefore acts like a silent poison. It destroys trust, weakens the interpersonal bond and undermines the healing power of contact.

2. Differentiation from related phenomena: Lack of empathy, burnout, cynicism

In order to clearly emphasise the special nature of indifference, it is necessary to distinguish it from related but not identical phenomena. Indifference is often confused with a lack of empathy. However, while a lack of empathy is often a constitutional or situational inability to empathise with the emotional situation of another, indifference usually implies a form of active avoidance. Indifference is not just a deficiency, but an attitude, a state of wilful or at least accepted uninvolvement. Those who are indifferent decide - consciously or habitually - not to allow themselves to be touched.

Burnout syndrome, which is particularly widespread in the medical field, must also be viewed in a differentiated way.

People who suffer from burnout are often emotionally exhausted, empty inside and no longer able to react adequately. Their emotional detachment is an expression of a state of overload and not a conscious lack of interest. Indifference, on the other hand, can also arise independently of exhaustion. It often manifests itself as a strategic or habitual reaction to systemic stress and can go hand in hand with functional performance. In medical professions in particular, where emotional distance is confused with professionalism, indifference often disguises itself as necessary objectivity.

Another related but independent phenomenon is cynicism. Cynicism is a form of disillusionment in which moral or human ideals are openly mocked or relativised. While indifference is usually silent, cynicism is articulated loudly, provocatively and often aggressively. Nevertheless, there is a close connection between the two: indifference can serve as a breeding ground for cynicism when emotional blunting turns into a dismissive attitude towards humanity . The transition is fluid. The transition is fluid. In clinical reality, it is not uncommon to see a disastrous interplay between the two attitudes, which systematically impedes empathic encounters.

3. Indifference as a moral failure or functional strategy?

The moral evaluation of indifference is ambivalent. On the one hand, it is seen as an expression of an ethical deficit: Anyone who is indifferent to a suffering person not only violates an interpersonal norm, but also undermines the foundation of any helping activity. Especially in the healing professions, whose ethos is based on care, concern and shared responsibility, indifference is hardly compatible with the professional ethos. It becomes a silent betrayal of one's own role, a kind of inner rupture between professional standards and lived reality.

On the other hand, indifference can also be understood as a functional strategy that serves to protect against emotional overload. Particularly in highly stressful fields of work, where pain, suffering, death and existential borderline experiences have to be dealt with on a daily basis, a certain form of emotional damping can be essential for survival. It enables distance, clarity and the ability to act where emotional involvement could paralyse or overwhelm. In this light, indifference does not appear to be a moral failure, but rather an adaptive reaction to chronic overload.

But even if indifference is seen as a protective mechanism, the question remains as to its long-term effects. What stabilises in the short term can destroy relationships in the long term, undermine trust and create moral numbness.

Such a functionalisation of indifference runs the risk of permanently damaging the ethical sensorium. Temporary distancing can turn into a habitual lack of involvement, necessary self-limitation into permanent avoidance of others. Indifference then loses its function and becomes a problem in itself.

4. The ethical relevance of emotional apathy in the medical profession

In no other professional field does indifference have such serious consequences as in medicine. Those who dedicate themselves to caring for others bear a special moral responsibility - not only for the physical well-being of their patients, but also for their emotional safety, their dignity and their subjective experience of illness. Indifference in the medical context is therefore not only an individual lack of compassion, but also an ethically relevant breach of the professional ideal. It jeopardises the basis of every therapeutic relationship, undermines the patient's trust and thwarts the intention of healing.

At the same time, the normative expectations of medical staff must remain realistic. No one can act with maximum empathy on a permanent basis without failing at their own limits. However, the ethical demand is not for permanent emotional availability, but for a willingness to encounter, to make a serious endeavour to meet the other person as a person. Indifference is problematic where it becomes an attitude - where it is no longer an expression of situational overload, but part of the professional self-image. Then medicine not only loses its ethical integrity, but also its healing power.

5. Philosophical concepts of indifference and their significance for medicine

Indifference has also been thematised in different contexts in philosophy. In the Stoic tradition, it was considered a virtue: indifference to external circumstances should lead to inner freedom. What people cannot influence should not affect them. However, this form of indifference had an introspective, self-centred character and was never related to interpersonal relationships. In modern contexts, on the other hand, indifference appears as an expression of moral apathy or as a symptom of a dehumanised society.

In her works, Hannah Arendt described the "banality of evil" as a form of thoughtless indifference in which people become part of inhuman systems without pausing to reflect. In this perspective, indifference is not an active desire for evil, but the passive acceptance of injustice - an ethical blindness that arises from habit, adaptation or indifference. This analysis is highly relevant to medicine. For here too, indifference is often not malicious neglect, but an unconscious routine, an adaptation to a system that does not reward attention.

In existentialist concepts, on the other hand, indifference is seen as an escape from freedom, as a refusal to take responsibility for one's own decisions. Those who are indifferent make themselves the object of circumstances and withdraw from ethical reflection. In medicine, this attitude can be dangerous: It absolves you of responsibility, numbs your conscience and trivialises the consequences of your own actions. It is therefore all the more important not to regard indifference as a neutral state, but as a morally and existentially significant phenomenon - with far-reaching consequences for medical action.

Chapter 3: When routine becomes a trap- mechanisms of blunting

1. Everyday life in the clinic and practice: routines as structure and stress

Everyday clinical practice is characterised by a large number of recurring processes. Whether it's ward rounds, taking blood samples, administering medication, documentation, informative discussions or administrative tasks - the working day in medical facilities is largely structured by routines. These routines primarily serve to stabilise and organise a highly complex system. They enable standardisation, reduce sources of error and create a degree of predictability that can be crucial, particularly in time-critical or emergency medical situations. Routines are therefore not only a tool for increasing efficiency, but also a protective mechanism against being overwhelmed by complexity.

However, precisely because routine takes on a relieving function, it harbours a high risk: it can lead to a creeping alienation in which the dynamics of interpersonal encounters are masked by automated action. In the repetitive execution of standardised processes, the exceptional becomes the exception, the human becomes a disturbance, the individual becomes a burden. The significance of the individual moment is replaced by the expectation that everything will be the same as always. The patient is no longer perceived as a unique subject, but as a representative of a pattern, as the bearer of a clinical image, as part of an organisational process.

This mechanisation of perception is not a moral weakness, but the result of a system that is geared towards efficiency, documentation and scalability. In such a system, time is a scarce commodity, attention is a limited factor and emotional involvement is a potential disruptive factor. Anyone who interacts with dozens of patients every day must protect themselves, set boundaries and learn to organise interpersonal encounters in a functional way. But the danger lies precisely in this self-protection: it can turn into indifference without being consciously realised.

2. Cognitive and emotional effects of monotonous sequences of actions

The cognitive processes that take place under monotonous conditions have been well researched. Repetition leads to the development of automated patterns that help to save energy and react quickly to familiar patterns. This automation is an evolutionary principle that facilitates the rapid recognition of clinical pictures and standard procedures in everyday clinical practice. However, the more these automatisms take effect, the more individual judgement fades into the background. What appears familiar is no longer scrutinised, but covered up by routines. This applies not only to diagnostic judgements, but also to social interactions. The conversation with the patient becomes a ritual, the medical history a questionnaire, the ward round a list of points to be worked through.

On an emotional level, this automatisation leads to a reduction in affective resonance. The repeated confrontation with pain, fear, suffering and dying no longer evokes the same emotional depth as the first professional experiences. This development is not pathological per se, but initially a sign of professional detachment. However, the more this demarcation becomes entrenched, the greater the risk of emotional blunting. Empathic resonance gives way to functional disinterest, emotional sensitivity is replaced by an inner emptiness that can hardly be consciously perceived. This state is dangerous because it is not loud, not conspicuous and cannot be scandalised. It develops quietly, gradually, often unnoticed - and that is precisely why it is so powerful.

Those affected often only realise their change at a late stage. Signs such as a declining interest in conversations with patients, the shortening of interpersonal contacts, the reduction of closeness or the defence against complex emotional situations are the first signals of an inner withdrawal. Many do not perceive this state as a loss, but as a necessary distancing. However, this interpretation obscures the fact that it is not just a matter of building up protection, but of giving up participation - often permanently.

3. Automation of medical decisions and loss of compassion

The ongoing digitalisation of medicine has led to a profound change in the decision-making architecture. Diagnoses are increasingly based on algorithmic processes, treatment paths follow standardised guidelines and the assessment of clinical situations is supplemented or replaced by structured scoring systems. This development undoubtedly has advantages: it increases the traceability of medical decisions, promotes standardisation and reduces subjective errors. However, these advantages are accompanied by a fundamental loss - namely the transfer of medical responsibility to technical systems and the disappearance of human judgement as a moral factor.

When doctors' actions are based on technical plausibility and algorithmic specifications, a new form of diffusion of responsibility arises. Decisions appear objective, neutral, impersonal - they are no longer an expression of an ethically based devotion to the patient, but the result of a systemic output. The doctor thus becomes the executor of an external logic, the individual behind the clinical data set recedes into the background. Under such conditions, compassion appears to be disruptive: it costs time, creates doubt and thwarts efficiency.

This loss of empathy is not necessarily associated with open rejection or hostility. Much more frequently, it manifests itself in a "no longer wanting to be recognised", an inner turning away, a silent withdrawal from interpersonal encounters. Patients sense this state very clearly: they report "cold stares", "processing", the feeling of no longer being meant as a person. As a result, medicine loses a central part of its healing potential - not at the level of technology, but at the level of the relationship.

4. The role of time pressure, shift systems and economic targets

Time pressure is a key driver of indifference in the medical system. It not only reduces the duration, but also the quality of interpersonal interactions. Those who rush from appointment to appointment no longer perceive the dialogue with the patient as an opportunity, but as an obstacle. Looking at the clock replaces looking at the other person's face. This is reinforced by shift systems in which responsibility is fragmented, handovers remain incomplete and continuous relationships are impossible. The development of trusting relationships, which would be particularly important in difficult clinical situations, is structurally prevented.

Added to this is the economic pressure that weighs on medical facilities. Hospitals have to make a profit, doctors are measured by case numbers and nursing staff are under constant suspicion of inefficiency. In this climate, it is hardly possible to prioritise the needs of individual people over systemic requirements. Medical interaction becomes a transaction, attention becomes a negligible variable. In this context, indifference is not an individual decision, but the result of systematic dehumanisation.

5. How a sense of responsibility dissolves under routine conditions

Responsibility thrives on attentiveness, judgement and moral presence. However, under conditions of chronic overwork, routinised decision-making and a lack of personal feedback, this sense of responsibility threatens to fade. The relationship with the patient becomes fleeting, there is no feedback on decisions and the moral resonance chamber atrophies. Individuals lose the feeling that their actions have an ethical dimension - not because they are irresponsible, but because they work in an environment that fragments and neutralises responsibility.

The loss of a sense of responsibility manifests itself in small gestures: in the decision to ignore a critical value, not to enquire about a symptom, not to see a patient again. These are not spectacular lapses, but quiet omissions, the consequences of which often only become apparent in retrospect. Precisely because they are so unspectacular, they usually remain without consequences - and thus reproduce themselves undisturbed.

The moral dimension of routine lies in its ability to empty action without visibly changing it. The form remains the same, the content disappears. Those who work in this way for years not only lose contact with others, but also with themselves. Indifference then becomes the basic inner attitude - not because the person is bad, but because the system does not allow any other attitude without breaking.

Chapter 4: Structural causes of medical indifference

1. Healthcare systems under the primacy of economics

The increasing dominance of economic rationality in the healthcare sector has transformed medicine to an extent that goes far beyond technical and organisational changes. Where the medical profession used to be considered a vocation, characterised by humanistic ideals, a deeply rooted sense of responsibility towards the patient and an ethically based attitude, today a business-structured self-image has taken over in many cases. In this new paradigm, efficiency rather than care is at the centre of medical practice.

This economisation is not only expressed in language - for example in terms such as "treatment case", "bed disposition", "length of stay management" or "yield optimisation" - but also in concrete management instruments that have a deep impact on daily practice. Flat rates per case, performance recording sheets, budgeting systems and benchmark comparisons create incentives that serve the economic balance sheet rather than patient welfare. The result is a creeping devaluation of the individual. The patient is no longer seen as a suffering person, but as an economic factor - as a cost centre, potential source of income or statistical variable.

This change has a massive impact on the attitude of people working in medicine. Those who work in a system that does not provide for care will be less willing to give it in the long term. Compassion, attentiveness, patience and the ability to engage in dialogue will no longer be regarded as key skills, but as emotions that are difficult to calculate and potentially disruptive. People are excluded from the logic of care - not through explicit devaluation, but through structural ignorance. The result is a system that not only allows indifference, but actively produces it.

2. Staff shortages and excessive demands are the norm

In hardly any other professional field are overwork, chronic stress and exhaustion as widespread as in the medical sector. The staff shortage is not only the result of demographic developments or regional imbalances in care, but also largely an expression of political decisions, economic priorities and structural neglect. For decades, nursing professions have been underfunded, working conditions have deteriorated and medical activities have been burdened by increasing bureaucracy. The consequence is a care situation that can often only be maintained because staff are stretched beyond their limits.

This constant overload not only changes performance, but also the emotional climate. Those who work under time pressure, are constantly pushed to their limits and have no prospect of improvement inevitably develop protective mechanisms. These include emotional isolation, selective perception and a strong focus on what is immediately necessary. Humanity then becomes a luxury that we cannot afford. The capacity for empathic resonance atrophies, not because it is lacking, but because it no longer fits into the reality of everyday life.

The situation is particularly dramatic in nursing care, where the lack of time means that the most basic needs of patients - such as attention, personal hygiene and personal contact - can only be met in a rudimentary way. Many carers experience this as a permanent burden of conscience. However, when they see that commitment is not recognised, overtime is not paid and extra work is taken for granted, they react with emotional withdrawal. This withdrawal is not an expression of a moral deficit, but the result of structural violence - a violence that does not beat, but demoralises.

3. Bureaucracy, documentation requirements and digital interfaces

The idea that documentation serves quality assurance has led to a paradox in modern medicine: The more that is documented, the less time there is for the encounter. Digital patient files, medication lists, progress logs, form systems, data protection requirements and coding obligations tie up a considerable amount of working time - up to fifty per cent in some areas. Documentation is often not tailored to clinical reality, but rather to billing logic and legal protection. Doctors and nurses therefore increasingly feel like agents of a system that serves itself rather than the patient.

Increasing mechanisation is exacerbating this problem. Digital interfaces structure the clinical view: The monitor replaces the person, the cursor replaces the dialogue. Clinical reality becomes a grid of parameters, scores and checkboxes. Anything that does not fit into the predefined fields is lost from view. The encounter with the real person becomes a minor matter. Yet it is precisely this encounter that would be the prerequisite for successful therapy, for trust, for compliance and for healing in the broadest sense.

This digital transformation of medical interaction creates a twofold alienation: on the one hand, patients feel that they are no longer perceived as people, and on the other hand, medical professionals experience that their profession is increasingly disintegrating into technocratic duties. The feeling of no longer being effective in the true sense of the word leads to a loss of meaning and emotional emptying - both key prerequisites for the emergence of indifferent attitudes.

4. False incentives in the remuneration of medical services

In many countries, the remuneration of medical services is based on points systems, procedure catalogues or diagnosis codes. These systems set incentives that are not primarily based on medical or ethical needs, but on economic considerations. Complex interventions, technical services and instrument-based diagnostics are highly remunerated, while talking medicine, detailed medical histories, psychosocial discussions or palliative care are hardly taken into account. This asymmetry reflects a structural devaluation of dialogue, relationships and emotional work in medicine.

These disincentives have a subtle but lasting effect. Doctors are faced with the choice of either being economically successful or following their ethical intuition - it is often not possible to do both at the same time. Those who are considered empathetic are often ridiculed in teams. Those who take their time risk economic losses. Those who linger where others pass by delay the operational flow. This creates a culture of acceleration, compression, technical superiority - and emotional emptiness. In this system, indifference is not a personal failure, but a form of structural adaptation.

At the same time, this economic distortion leads to an unequal distribution of medical attention. Complex patients who cannot be clearly categorised - such as the chronically ill, the mentally distressed, the elderly in nursing homes - receive less medical attention because they are less "cost-effective". This system of indirect discrimination usually remains invisible because it is not based on individual decisions but on collectively internalised incentive systems.

5. Organisational coldness: Hospitals as companies instead of places of healing

For centuries, hospitals were regarded as special places: as spaces of care, concentration and healing. Even if they were not free of power and hierarchy, human need was at the centre of the architectural, social and symbolic order. This function has changed over time. Today, management concepts, lean processes, personnel controlling, business plans and facility management dominate. Administration has taken over the primacy in many buildings and decisions are based on key figures rather than values.

This functional logic not only permeates the organisation, but also shapes the culture. What counts is the conservation of resources, not the quality of the relationship. What is sought is a smooth process, not a successful dialogue. What is rewarded is speed, not pause. In such an environment, care, patience and moral presence become resistance to the logic of the system. Those who cling to this risk isolation, excessive demands or professional failure.

This coldness is not loud, not brutal, not openly violent - but it is effective. It creates a climate in which human impulses only appear to be a risk, in which ethics become a minor matter and in which indifference mutates into a rational consequence. The hospital as a place of healing does not die through external destruction, but through the creeping revaluation of its inner principles. When the organisation becomes a machine, all that remains for the human is a place on the margins - as a sentimental relic, not as a lived reality.

Chapter 5: The invisible victims- when the person behind the case disappears

1. The view through the case number: depersonalisation in patient care

In modern medical practice, the management of patients is highly structured by technical, logistical and billing-related categories. The patient no longer appears as a person with a history, emotions and needs, but as the bearer of an administratively manageable case. The case number replaces the name, the residence status the life context, the diagnosis the individual horizon of experience. This form of depersonalisation is usually not carried out with hostile intentions, but as a result of structural necessities arising from efficiency considerations, time pressure and administrative requirements. However, the consequences are serious.

This shift in perspective turns the patient into a function within a system. Their individuality is translated into standardised procedures, their subjective distress is transformed into objective parameters. The question of how they feel, what they fear and how they experience their illness gives way to the question of how they should be categorised within the existing case structure. What counts is not who the patient is, but what is to be done with them. In medical documentation, these tendencies are reflected in the form of standardised findings, text module-based progress descriptions and formalised doctor's letters, in which the personal is no longer visible.

This depersonalisation has an impact on the relationship: doctors no longer see people as unique counterparts, but as representatives of a standardised case. The danger lies in the fact that actions are no longer determined by encounters, but by categorisation. In such a framework, compassion is difficult to maintain because it requires a closeness that is systematically prevented by administrative grids. The result is a silent impoverishment of the medical relationship - functional, factual, indifferent.

2. Subtle violence through ignorance, lack of time and disregard

The indifference that arises from this structural depersonalisation rarely manifests itself in open forms. It is not loud, not brutal, not deliberate. Its violence is subtle - and that is precisely why it is so profound. It manifests itself in the absence of glances, in unanswered questions, in routine actions without announcement, in the wordless performance of unpleasant procedures, in the omission of personal address, in silence in the face of fear. It is a violence of disregard, of silent distance, of consistently ignoring the human subject.

Patients who are exposed to this indifference experience their existence as devalued. They report that they feel like "a piece of meat", like "a number", like "an obstacle in the process". These statements are more than just metaphors. They testify to a deep alienation in which one's own subjectivity is no longer reflected. The sick person, who is already in a state of physical and psychological vulnerability, is cared for in an atmosphere in which they do not feel seen, heard or recognised. The patient's already fragile identity is shattered by the coldness he is met with - not through rejection, but through disinterest.

This form of subtle violence is barely recognised in the system. It cannot be measured, documented or expressed in figures. It happens in the space in between - where language is silenced, where closeness is denied, where humanity is withdrawn. In a system that is primarily focussed on visible mistakes, this form of violation remains invisible. But it leaves its mark - deep, barely healable wounds in the patient's soul.

3. Psychological stress due to symptoms that are not taken seriously

One particularly harmful aspect of structural indifference is the devaluation of the patient's subjective perception. Anyone who describes complaints that cannot be clearly measured or substantiated by diagnostic equipment runs the risk of not being taken seriously. This phenomenon particularly affects patients with chronic pain, functional disorders, psychosomatic complaints or complex, diffuse symptoms. Their stories do not fit the mould of medical clarity, they contradict the logic of a quick diagnosis, they require patience, listening and empathy.

In a system based on time optimisation and diagnostic efficiency, these patients are "difficult". They demand attention without a clear diagnosis. They bring with them questions to which there are no simple answers. And they call into question the medical self-image, which is based on objectifiability and evidence. The reaction of the system is often rejection, trivialisation or silence. The patient feels as if they are a nuisance, oversensitive, labelled as mentally disturbed. Their perception is relativised, their complaints devalued, their subjectivity delegitimised.

The psychological strain this causes is considerable. If you don't feel seen, taken seriously or validated, you start to doubt yourself. Self-perception collapses under the weight of professional ignorance. Fear turns into shame, insecurity into despair. Many of these patients develop secondary psychological disorders - depression, anxiety disorders, social withdrawal phenomena. Others seek support in alternative healing methods, in radical self-diagnoses or in mistrust of the entire healthcare system. In these cases, medical indifference has a double effect: not only does it fail to provide help, it also causes additional damage.

4. The fatal dynamic between medical indifference and patient mistrust

In a society in which access to medical knowledge is no longer exclusive, in which patients inform themselves before, during and after contact with doctors via the internet, social media and patient forums, trust is an increasingly fragile resource. This trust depends not only on professional expertise, but above all on the experience of being recognised and respected as a human being. In this context, indifference acts like a poison that slowly but surely creeps into the relationship.

Patients who experience indifference begin to doubt - not just the person, but the institution. Isolated unease turns into structural mistrust. This mistrust has far-reaching consequences: It leads to refusal of therapy, changes of doctor, conflicts, aggression, belief in conspiracies and an erosion of social acceptance of medical authority. The public debate about medical behaviour, the growing criticism of conventional medicine, the popularity of alternative treatment methods - all this is not only an expression of ideological differences, but often also a reaction to real experiences of medical alienation.

The fatal dynamic between medical indifference and patient mistrust is a cycle that stabilises itself: The more indifferent the system acts, the more distrustful the patients become. The more distrustful the patients become, the more the practitioners withdraw - out of self-protection, defence and excessive demands. This withdrawal, in turn, is experienced by the patients as renewed coldness - and reinforces the mistrust. In this cycle, the medical relationship is in danger of losing its dialogue structure. What remains is interaction without relationship, communication without trust, care without encounter.

5. Reports from the field: voices of patients and relatives

Numerous reports from patients and relatives impressively show how hurtful medical indifference is experienced. A young woman with chronic pain describes how she was repeatedly told not to behave like that. An elderly man reports that nobody spoke to him when he cried after a diagnosis. A mother describes how her seriously ill son was moved to another corridor without explanation and without her knowing why. These reports are not spectacular, not scandalising - but they are honest, haunting and harrowing.

What unites them is the feeling of not being recognised as a human being. It is not the lack of medication, not the mistakes in treatment, not the lack of technology that makes these experiences so painful - but the lack of attention. The experience that nobody was interested. That no one asked what you needed, what you felt, what you hoped for or feared. It is this void - the void of attention - that deepens suffering, increases pain and escalates fear.

Such reports are more than just isolated cases. They are an expression of a structural problem that cannot be solved by quality management, process optimisation or patient surveys. They show that medical care without human contact is not only incomplete, but also dangerous. Because it leaves people alone - where they are most vulnerable.

Chapter 6: Silent brutalisation - indifference as a social phenomenon in a team

1. Group dynamics in medical hierarchies

The social architecture of medical facilities is characterised by pronounced hierarchies, both formal and informal. Medical ranks, nursing structures, disciplinary responsibilities and institutional demarcations form a system based on clear roles. Within this structure, specific power relationships, rules of conduct and unspoken expectations emerge that not only organise daily interaction, but also have a profound influence on it. Group behaviour in the medical environment is therefore not just collegial cooperation, but an interaction space characterised by social mechanisms that create, stabilise and control norms.

This dynamic harbours great risks for the development of indifference as a collective attitude. This is because social adaptation processes are particularly intense within medical teams. If you want to belong, you not only have to prove yourself professionally, but also emotionally. This often means putting aside one's own doubts, feelings or ethical dissonances in favour of consistent team behaviour. The informal rules - "this is how we do it here", "you have to stand over it", "that's just everyday life" - characterise the moral climate just as much as guidelines or laws.

Those starting out in their careers in particular experience this dynamic as a profound challenge. Their original attitude - characterised by idealism, compassion and ethical standards - comes under pressure early on. They observe that experienced colleagues keep their distance, forego emotions and insist on efficiency. Those who do not adapt risk social isolation, subtle devaluation or even open criticism. This is how a gradual process of adaptation begins: moral intuition turns into inner withdrawal, empathetic willingness into functional behaviour. The group moulds the individual - not through conviction, but through silent pressure.

2. Cynicism as a collective protective wall against emotional overload

Cynicism is a widespread reaction to chronic overload, institutional stagnation and moral exhaustion. In medical teams, it often develops as an expression of deeply felt frustration. When the system is overloaded, when patient fates are repeated at high frequency, when one's own ideals are regularly shattered by reality, then emotional defence becomes a survival strategy. Cynicism enables distance, protects against closeness, preserves functioning. Irony, mockery, resignation: these are all signs of self-protection that is not based on coldness, but on pain.

As a collective attitude, cynicism is particularly effective. It connects, stabilises and creates a sense of togetherness among the burdened. A shared suffering is expressed in a humorous form, which would otherwise remain speechless. But the price is high. Because cynicism is not neutral. It changes perception. It moulds language. It distorts reality. Patients are no longer seen as people in need, but as annoying cases, as overburdened clients, as "the ones from room 12". Relatives become "the annoying ones", complex cases become "the psychos". What was once considered an exception is becoming a basic attitude: emotional shutdown, contempt for need, defence against compassion.

In this atmosphere, every empathic impulse is relativised by collective devaluation. Laughing at a suffering patient, a sarcastic comment on a child's fear, a mocking look at a death - they seem like harmless relief at first. But they have a lasting effect on the climate. Cynicism is a psychological sedative with side effects: It provides short-term relief, but destroys ethical resilience in the long term.

3. Silence, complicity and the disappearance of moral responsibility

The dominant attitudes and behavioural patterns in teams go beyond simple imitation. They create a normative order that dictates what can be said, what must be kept quiet and what is taboo. In such social fields, silence is a central element in maintaining power. It stabilises existing imbalances, protects established routines and prevents change. Those who remain silent evade responsibility - but also the possibility of acting ethically.

Silence in the face of borderline or openly hurtful behaviour is particularly problematic. A derogatory tone with patients, the deliberate ignoring of needs, a sarcastic comment about mentally ill people - all of this can be part of everyday life without ever being openly addressed. The reactions to this follow a familiar pattern: you look away, carry on, distance yourself inwardly but remain outwardly conformist. The moral impulse to intervene is suppressed - not out of indifference, but out of fear of conflict, of marginalisation, of going it alone without support.

This dynamic leads to a collective erosion of moral responsibility. Responsibility becomes diffuse, invisible, dissolved into competences. Everyone is "just doing their job". The suffering of the patient becomes a side effect of the organisation, not an object of personal concern. This creates a system in which ethical behaviour is no longer expected because it is not systematically protected. Looking the other way becomes the ethos - not explicitly, but perceptibly. Those who look away risk standing alone.

4. Social sanctions against empathetic colleagues

Although empathy is officially desirable in medical discourse, it is often undesirable in everyday practice. Those who behave empathetically often come under pressure. The empathic colleague disrupts the process, demands more time, asks uncomfortable questions, awakens emotions that the team has long since suppressed. They remind you of what you have given up: closeness, listening, ethical struggle. In a functional system, this reminder is uncomfortable - it is fended off, suppressed or ironised.

This defence rarely happens openly, but via subtle social mechanisms: the empathetic colleague is excluded from conversations, mocking remarks are made about her "idealism", she is no longer involved in decision-making processes or she is symbolically "burnt out" by being assigned the most emotionally demanding patients. The social pressure is quiet but massive. Those who do not comply risk being ostracised - not formally, but tangibly.

This experience is particularly stressful for young doctors. They experience the conflict between ethical standards and systemic reality as existential. Many experience inner crises, consider leaving the profession, switch to other sectors or develop cynical defence mechanisms to protect themselves. In this way, the system loses the people it actually urgently needs: the compassionate, the thoughtful, the ethically vigilant.

5. Culture of looking the other way: when misbehaviour becomes the norm

Perhaps the most serious effect of indifferent team cultures is the normalisation of misconduct. What was considered morally unacceptable becomes the accepted standard through constant repetition and collective silence. This normalisation is unspectacular, creeping, silent. It is not heralded by a dramatic break - but by many small, almost imperceptible shifts in boundaries. A patient is shouted at and nobody says anything. A dying person is left alone and everyone goes home. A colleague openly expresses contempt and no one objects.

The more frequently such situations occur, the more the moral sense evaporates. What remains is a functional system that is geared towards stability, not humanity. This stability has a price: it creates indifference as a structural norm. Anyone who violates it causes unrest in the system. And therefore not only is misbehaviour tolerated, but compassion is repressed. The organisation does not protect the ethos, but the process. Humanity is no longer a goal, but a disruption.

In such a culture, ethical resistance is only possible with difficulty. It seems irrational, inefficient and disruptive. And yet it is necessary - because without it, the medical system loses its legitimacy. Where turning a blind eye becomes the rule, conscience dies. And where conscience is silent, brutalisation begins. Not loudly, not visibly, not violently - but fatally.

Chapter 7: Training without attitude? The role of medical teaching

1. Academisation versus humanity: curricula without empathy training

The development of medical teaching into a scientific-academic system was historically necessary and in many respects also a step forward. It brought medicine out of the realm of speculative medicine and into the sphere of scientific methodology and empirical evidence. Today, however, there is a worrying imbalance: while scientific content is taught precisely and in great depth during training, the human dimension of medical practice is largely ignored. Medicine has become academic - but in many places it is in the process of losing its character as a healing, compassionate profession.

The curricular structure reflects this shift. The majority of medical studies consist of biological, chemical, physical, pathophysiological and pharmacological content. In contrast, human communication, psychosocial concepts of illness, emotional dynamics or ethical conflicts appear to be marginalised learning content - if they occur systematically at all. And even where they are included in the curriculum, there is often a lack of space for genuine dialogue, personal development and emotional feedback.

In addition, there is a basic attitude that resonates latently in many faculties: that empathy is a matter of personality, which one may or may not have - but not a competence that can be specifically promoted, protected and cultivated. This assumption is not only empirically incorrect, but also dangerous. It leaves education in an ethical vacuum in which students are left to their own devices when it comes to questions of inner attitude. Those who study in such a functionalised system learn a lot about illness - but little about being human in illness. The indifference that is so frequently encountered in everyday clinical practice begins here - in the systematic concealment of the emotional reality of medical action.

2. Examination culture, grade pressure and the decoupling of theory and practice

The logic of medical training increasingly follows the principles of a standardised meritocracy. Examinations are extensive, highly frequent and strictly formalised. Students have to memorise large amounts of information in the shortest possible time, the relevance of which is often incomprehensible in everyday clinical practice. The examination becomes an end in itself. The content no longer serves the formation of medical awareness, but rather the mastery of a rigid selection system.

The effects of this examination logic on the attitude of future doctors are considerable. There is hardly any time for reflection, doubt, personal development or ethical debate. Everything that is not relevant to the examination seems secondary - and therefore also everything that concerns the human aspect: self-reflection, understanding the patient's world, developing a mindful relationship culture. This reduction to the functional, retrievable and technical creates a perception of medicine that is cognitively sharp but emotionally blind.

The disconnect between theory and actual practice is particularly problematic. In many stages of training, learning takes place in an artificial world - in lecture theatres, on tables, in collections of questions - while the reality of medical practice makes completely different demands: Listening, enduring, communicating, making decisions in the face of uncertainty, accompanying the dying. There is often hardly any connection between these worlds. Students learn to reproduce facts, but not to situate themselves in professional behaviour. They can differentiate, but not interpret. They can name, but not encounter. This gap creates an inner void in which indifference can flourish - not as an attitude of disinterest, but as a result of a lack of integration between knowledge and reality.

3. Early indoctrination into a system of efficiency and objectivity

Even in their first semesters, medical students learn that efficiency, distance and professionalism are central virtues of the medical profession. The ideal of professionalism is often equated with coolness, objectivity and imperturbability. Those who act too emotionally are seen as insecure, unstable or inefficient. The institution thus conveys an image of the doctor who is knowledgeable but not touched; who appears capable but not vulnerable; who acts but does not really meet. This moulding is profound - it does not take effect through formal teaching, but through the implicit curriculum: through role models, non-verbal signals, institutional routines.

Practical training, especially in the clinical sections, reinforces this development. Students are introduced to a system that is under massive time pressure, chronic staff shortages and high structural stress. They experience how senior physicians work through ward rounds every minute, how nursing staff reach their limits and how nobody really listens any more. And they quickly learn that if you want to survive, you have to work. Anyone who shows attention is slowed down. If you stand still, you disrupt the flow.

These early experiences leave their mark. Many young doctors lose their emotional openness during these first practical years. Not out of indifference, but out of survival instinct. They protect themselves by closing themselves off. They rationalise their behaviour because no one else sets an example. They adapt to a system that does not prepare them, but moulds them. And so begins the silent transformation that characterises so many reports from students and junior doctors: the loss of an inner orientation, the abandonment of an empathic ideal that is gradually replaced by distance. Here, indifference is not the result of a decision - but the result of an education system that does not teach an attitude.

4. Empathy as a "soft skill" or an indispensable competence?

In medical rhetoric, empathy is considered a desirable addition. It appears in mission statements, in patient brochures, in quality standards - but rarely at the centre of professional learning. Its categorisation as a "soft skill" suggests that it is a soft, optional ability that is only incidental to the hard core of the medical art. This categorisation is fatal. It undermines the understanding of what constitutes medical practice at its core.

Empathy is not an emotional extra. It is the prerequisite for understanding. Only those who can empathise with others can understand the meaning of symptoms, recognise the breaks in the life story and hear what is being said between the words. Without empathy, the medical view is blind to the subjective - and therefore to half of reality. At the same time, empathy is the key to successful communication, to increasing adherence, to reducing misunderstandings and errors. Devaluing it as a "soft factor" reveals a structural disregard for the anthropological depth of medicine.

The consequences of this disregard are visible: doctors who have not learnt how to deal with compassion feel defenceless. They develop defence mechanisms, rationalise, withdraw or perceive compassion as a threat to their ability to act. What is missing is systematic training in the question: How can you be empathetic without losing yourself? How can you allow closeness without burning out? How can you stay emotionally present without jeopardising your own stability? These questions are rarely asked - and therefore many medical biographies remain thrown back on themselves, without inner security, without emotional stability.

5. Approaches for an ethical-emotional educational reform in medical training

Humane medicine needs humane education. It needs teaching that not only imparts knowledge, but also develops an attitude. That prepares students not for exams, but for relationships. Teaching not only symptoms, but also meanings. Such a reform must start at several levels: curricular, institutional, cultural.

In curricular terms, this means that empathy, ethics, communication and self-reflection must not be treated as marginal topics, but as integral components of the degree programme - from the first semester onwards, not just in the compulsory electives. We need seminars in which values are discussed. Spaces in which uncertainty is allowed. Formats in which powerlessness, closeness, guilt and doubt can be openly discussed. And it needs people who can hold these spaces - not as lecturers, but as companions, as personalities, as medical role models.

Institutionally, reform means that organisations must have the courage to embed humanity not just rhetorically, but structurally. That time for reflection is not considered a luxury, but a necessity. That students are not only judged on their performance, but also on their attitude. That care is not devalued as weakness, but as an expression of professionalism.

Finally, culturally, it means that the medical self-image must change: Away from the myth of invulnerability, towards a realistic, human image of the doctor - as both a knower and a doubter, as both a doer and a listener, as both a professional and a sympathiser. Only then can the indifference that so often begins in medical training be transformed into a new form of attention: an attitude that sees the person before it acts.

Chapter 8: Indifference as a protective mechanism- Necessary or dangerous?

1. Psychological protection strategies in high-stress professions

Medical practice is characterised by a special constellation: doctors and nursing staff encounter people in exceptional existential situations on a daily basis. They are confronted with pain, fear, despair, hopelessness and death. At the same time, they themselves are under great pressure to perform, bear immense responsibility and have to make momentous decisions in a short space of time. This emotional and cognitive overload calls for psychological protection mechanisms that enable them to act without breaking down inside.

These protective mechanisms include rationalisation, cognitive detachment, depersonalisation of the other person, humour, sarcasm, suppression of work and a strong retreat to the professional. In clinical psychology, these phenomena are described as coping strategies that provide short-term relief but can lead to inner emptiness in the long term. Paradoxically, they are often most pronounced in helping professions - not because those affected are numb, but because they were originally particularly empathetic.

These protective mechanisms develop gradually, often unnoticed. They do not arise out of conviction, but out of necessity. Those who are confronted with severe suffering on a daily basis and at the same time have no opportunity to process it unconsciously look for ways to maintain their own equilibrium. The indifference that arises from this is a protective armour: an attempt to remain capable of acting without going under emotionally. It is not an expression of coldness, but of pain that has not been allowed to find expression.

2. The boundary between self-protection and emotional coldness

As helpful as protective mechanisms may be in the short term, they harbour the danger of taking on a life of their own in the long term. What begins as temporary distancing can develop into a permanent state of emotional isolation. The boundary between professional detachment and emotional coldness is fluid, difficult to recognise and varies from person to person.

A first indication of this crossing of boundaries is the change in language. Patients are no longer referred to as people, but as "cases", "numbers", "diagnoses" or "rooms". Their individuality is replaced by categories, their stories by abbreviations, their feelings by functional terms. Communication is also changing: sentences are becoming shorter, conversations more technical, eye contact less frequent, touching more functional. The relationship is reduced to what is necessary - the human element takes a back seat.

Another indicator is the loss of inner resonance. Situations that used to be touching - such as a death, a farewell, crying - no longer trigger any emotion. Your own vulnerability has disappeared. You don't notice it immediately - but at some point you realise that you no longer feel anything. This state is dangerous. Not because it is wrong or evil - but because it shows that psychological balance is no longer maintained through reflection, but through repression. It is a mental anaesthetic - necessary, but threatening if it becomes permanent.

3. Empathy as a risk: emotional exhaustion through closeness

Empathy is a central element of healing relationships - but it is also an emotional resource that can be exhausted. Those who empathise with people share their feelings, their fears and their insecurities. This is a highly demanding psychological endeavour. It requires not only openness, but also regulation, processing and self-reference. If these are not possible, empathy becomes a burden.

In medical care, this leads to a typical dilemma: those who get involved risk exhaustion. Those who isolate themselves risk indifference. Many medical professionals oscillate between these poles for years without finding a stable balance.

Professional groups with a high level of emotional closeness are particularly at risk - for example in palliative care, paediatric oncology, emergency care, psychiatry or intensive care.

This emotional exhaustion can manifest itself in various symptoms: sleep disorders, inner emptiness, withdrawal, cynicism, psychosomatic complaints, concentration problems or the loss of a sense of purpose. Secondary cynicism often develops, which serves to rationalise the increasing emotional numbness. People begin to make fun of patients, distance themselves linguistically and trivialise their own role - not out of arrogance, but out of a need for protection.

These processes are understandable, but also dangerous: they lead to a gradual loss of identity, in which one's own medical or nursing role is no longer experienced as meaningful. The person functions - but no longer lives inwardly.

4. The role of promoting resilience in professional self-care

Resilience - understood as the ability not only to endure stress, but to remain capable of acting within it - is a key resource in the medical context. However, it does not develop by itself. It is not an individual talent, but the result of personal competence, organisational support and cultural recognition. If you want to remain resilient, you need a stable professional environment in which compassion does not become a danger.

Resilience includes self-observation, self-care, emotional regulation, healthy boundaries, peer feedback and the ability to seek help in stressful situations. These skills can and must be learnt. But in many medical systems, there is a lack of structured programmes to develop them. There are hardly any spaces for supervision, hardly any time for collegial dialogue about ethical burdens, hardly any institutional culture of pausing to reflect. Instead, there is an implicit expectation that people will "get on with it".

Yet the opposite is necessary. Medical institutions should actively promote resilience: through mandatory reflection formats, ethical case discussions, integrated supervision, a transparent culture of error, humane leadership and by enabling grief, doubt and personal expression. Only where there is room for emotions can indifference as a protective reaction be avoided. And only where people learn how to protect themselves without hurting others can a professional culture of humanity emerge.

5. Possibilities of demarcation without ethical withdrawal

Demarcation is not a betrayal of medical or nursing ethics. It is a necessary component of professional behaviour. But it must be done consciously, reflectively and responsibly.

Demarcation does not mean turning away - it means maintaining the boundary between you and me without devaluing you. It is about staying in contact with suffering without letting it engulf you.

This form of behaviour can be described as "resonant distance" or "connected self-limitation". It allows closeness without overwhelming. It keeps compassion alive without tipping over into pity. It preserves professionalism without becoming cold. Developing this attitude requires self-awareness, regular self-reflection and a continuous commitment to one's own professional ethos.

A central component of this attitude is the ability to differentiate within oneself: recognising one's own limits, recognising internal warning signals early on and consciously asking for support. It is equally important to allow grief, share burdens and openly name powerlessness. Those who can talk about what moves them stay in motion. Those who repress lose resonance.

In addition, a culture is needed in which humanity is seen as a strength - not an obstacle. In which empathy is rewarded - not sanctioned. In which the medical attitude is not measured by output, but by the quality of the relationship. Only in such a culture can indifference be overcome - not through moral appeals, but by structurally enabling an attitude that protects humanity without breaking it.

Chapter 9: When systems become blunt- institutional indifference as an expression of structural failure

1. From attitude to structure: How organisations create indifference

Institutional indifference is more than the sum of individual indifference. It arises where the structure of an organisation itself becomes the bearer of an attitude - namely an attitude of systematic disinterest towards subjective experiences, individual needs and moral tensions. In medical institutions, this attitude manifests itself not only through a lack of attention, but also through the absence of resonance spaces in which the humanity of the actions could be perceived at all. In this way, indifference is no longer experienced as a personal weakness, but as an inescapable part of institutional reality.

This structural decoupling of organisation and ethics is particularly dangerous because it is often not consciously reflected upon. Organisations act in a supposedly "value-neutral" manner because they rely on processes, guidelines and standardisation. But this is precisely where the danger lies: to the extent that the moral is no longer considered a relevant element of organisational self-description, the institutional reference to the patient as a person is also lost. The system no longer reflects the fact that we are dealing with human suffering, existential fragility and morally highly charged situations. The organisation becomes an administrative unit for biological-technical processes, not the bearer of ethical responsibility.

This form of indifference is so powerful because it is transferred to the individual. Employees intuitively sense that their moral impulses have no place in the system. The structure acts like a filter through which ethical commitment can neither become visible nor effective. The result is a silent resignation that is not caused by individual decisions, but by the long-term experience that one's own compassion is structurally irrelevant.

2. The logic of the system: efficiency, control, standardisation

Modern medicine is subject to the imperative of optimisation. Quality management, process control, time management, key performance indicator systems, benchmarking and certification procedures determine everyday clinical practice. These instruments are not bad per se - they can minimise errors, create transparency and distribute resources better. However, their one-sided dominance fundamentally changes the character of the medical organisation : what counts is what can be calculated. What counts is what can be controlled. And what cannot be controlled - the spontaneous encounter, the unplanned conversation, the hesitation in the face of a difficult fate - becomes invisible.

This control logic creates a paradoxical dynamic. The more attempts are made to "secure" the organisation through specifications and standards, the more it loses its ability for human self-correction. Interpersonal signals - such as a care assistant's feeling that something is wrong even though the values are unremarkable - have no place in the system because they cannot be substantiated. The organisation no longer listens. It only reacts to what is measurable. This means that indifference is not the result of a lack of emotion, but the consequence of a structure that no longer needs emotion in order to function.

The systemic primacy of control entails a deprofessionalisation of the players. Roles are defined so narrowly by sets of rules, checklists and guidelines that individual intuition, moral creativity and personal responsibility are increasingly suppressed. The actor becomes an interface between the system and the case - no longer a morally embedded person who interacts with other people. This dehumanisation lies at the heart of institutional indifference.

3. The role of leadership and management culture

Leadership is not just decision-making competence - it is always also a cultural setting. Every manager shapes the moral climate of an organisation through their behaviour, their language, their priorities and what they allow or prevent. This role is particularly important in medical facilities. Because when working with sick, vulnerable and dying people, leadership that is purely focussed on efficiency can have serious ethical consequences.

You can recognise indifferent leadership not by the fact that it is explicitly inhumane - but by the fact that it systematically ignores the human element. It does not ask: "How are the employees doing?" It asks: "How much overtime is still acceptable?" It does not ask: "What does this decision mean for the treatment of patients?" It asks: "How will this affect capacity utilisation?" In this logic, humanity becomes a subordinate category, moral reflection a private matter. Responsibility is reduced to management - ethics becomes a side note.

The exact opposite would be necessary. Managers should see themselves as ethical leaders. They should not only enable performance, but also strengthen attitudes. Not just manage resources, but open up spaces for dialogue. Not just develop strategies, but convey meaning. Good leadership cannot be recognised by the number of key figures met, but by the depth of the conversations that take place around them. Where leadership is silent, the system talks. And the system does not recognise empathy.

4. Organisational blindness for the subjective

Organisations tend to reduce complexity. They have to decide what they consider relevant - and what not. Subjective experiences often fall through the cracks. They are not comparable, cannot be documented and cannot be translated into key figures. As a result, they are systematically devalued. Feelings are regarded as disturbing, moods as irrational, individual perceptions as unreliable. The organisation only "sees" what it can measure - and only "hears" what it expects.

This blindness to the subjective has far-reaching consequences. Patients no longer experience themselves as subjects, but as objects of medical measures. Employees no longer experience themselves as agents, but as fulfilers of externally determined requirements. The organisation no longer reacts to internal signals, but only to external control. It loses the ability for moral self-awareness - a state that can be described as ethical numbness.

This blindness cannot be overcome by more data or more complex algorithms. It can only be corrected through structural openness - through spaces in which subjective experiences are not only allowed, but also desired. Through formats in which feelings can be talked about without having to be immediately translated into action. Through a culture in which being human is not seen as a risk, but as a resource. Where this succeeds, the organisation begins to listen again - and with it the people who work in it.

5. Ways out of structural blunting

Structural indifference is a systemic phenomenon - and can therefore only be overcome systemically. It is not enough to appeal to the morals of individual actors. What is needed is an institutional change that not only tolerates human behaviour, but also protects it structurally. This first requires the admission that the system itself has become ill - not out of malice, but out of a one-sided orientation. This diagnosis is uncomfortable, but necessary.

Therapy begins with small, concrete steps: regular supervision sessions in which emotional stress is discussed; team meetings in which there is room for self-reflection; guidelines that integrate ethical issues instead of excluding them; decision-making processes that actively involve those affected. But structural reforms are also needed: personnel management that systematically takes care into account; controlling that not only measures performance, but also relationships; an understanding of quality that sees humanity not as an add-on, but as a target criterion.

Above all, however, we need a new idea of what a medical organisation is: not a machine park, not a billing system, not a production plant - but a social, ethical, living structure in which people act for people. If this idea becomes the guiding principle again, indifference can not only be avoided, but overcome. Not through more efficiency - but through more attention. Not through control - but through relationship. Not through instruction - but through attitude.

Chapter 10: Suffering without echo - the patients' perspective

1. The experience of being unseen during the course of the disease

For many people, the experience of being ill is a radical interruption to their everyday biography. What was previously taken for granted - physical integrity, self-determination, the ability to plan - begins to falter. Added to this is the feeling of being at the mercy of a world whose language, procedures and decision-making processes are initially unfamiliar. In this new world, patients search for orientation - and above all for recognition of their experiences. They don't just want to be treated, they want to be seen. Not just managed, but understood. Not just perceived as a medical case, but as a person with a history, values, relationships, fears and hopes.

The feeling of being unseen is often not caused by gross omissions, but by a multitude of small, seemingly insignificant interactions: not responding to a personal comment, ignoring emotional impulses, silently leaving the room, answering questions without making eye contact. The overall impression is one of fundamental devaluation. The patient no longer feels like the subject of their own medical history, but as an object in a process controlled by others.

This alienation becomes particularly painful when it drags on over a longer period of time. What is initially irritating becomes an inner certainty: I am not meant. Nobody is interested in my inner state. I am not part of a relationship, but part of a schedule. This state not only causes emotional pain, but also a loss of trust that can jeopardise the entire therapeutic relationship.

2. Speechlessness, isolation and the loss of subjectivity

In situations of illness, it is not only the body that changes, but also the ability to speak. Many people lack the words to express their experiences in stressful moments. They feel diffuse fears, existential worries, moral conflicts - but cannot find the words to express them. When they then encounter medical staff who are themselves involved in functional modes of speech, a double speechlessness arises. One side cannot speak, the other does not listen. The conversation falls silent - not because no one has anything to say, but because there is no space for real dialogue.

This speechlessness leads to isolation. Those who are not heard withdraw. Those who experience no response fall silent inside. What remains is a feeling of abandonment - in the midst of an environment that should actually be caring. This social isolation is often overlooked in medical discussions because it cannot be measured. It is not a symptom, a diagnosis or a code. But it is real. It eats into the experience of those affected, causing shame, insecurity and alienation.

This experience is particularly dramatic for people who are already socially vulnerable - such as the elderly, chronically ill or mentally distressed. They often experience the medical system not as saving them, but as closing them off. Their subjectivity - their thoughts, feelings, perspectives - is systematically marginalised. What remains is the body as a carrier of data - and the ego, which withdraws from the system because it can no longer find a place in it.

3. Violations through silence, avoidance and functional communication

Not only what is said, but also what is not said has an effect. In medicine in particular, silence often has immense power - a power that can heal or hurt. Remaining silent at a patient's bedside can create closeness. Leaving the room in silence can deepen isolation. It depends on the attitude - on what resonates in the silence: Interest or disinterest, presence or escape, openness or reticence.

Many patients report moments when they felt deeply hurt by the behaviour of medical staff - not because something was done, but because something was omitted. Not a look, not a word, not a pause. These micro-injuries add up to a feeling of systematic devaluation. You are not important enough to be spoken to. Not significant enough to be noticed. Not human enough to be touched.

Functional communication reinforces this impression. It is technically precise, but existentially empty. It explains what happens to the body, but not what it does to the person. It informs about risks, but not about hopes. It clarifies, but does not accompany. It is necessary - and yet insufficient. Because people don't just want to know what is happening. They also want to know that someone is there to accompany them. That they are not just the object of measures, but the subject of a compassionate gaze.

4. The search for meaning, comfort and support in the medical system

Confronting illness often raises existential questions. Why does it affect me? What does it mean for my life, for my relationships, for my faith? How do I deal with the loss of control, of future, of identity? These questions cannot be treated - but they can be heard. They don't need a solution, they need resonance. Not answers, but support.

However, many patients experience the opposite. Their questions are dismissed as irrational, their search for meaning as a minor matter, their grief as inefficient. They feel that there is no room for their inner experience - neither in the schedule, nor in the language, nor in the attitude of the institution. The medical system thus becomes a place where they are helped physically but abandoned emotionally.

Yet it is precisely here that a space would be possible that goes far beyond medical help. A space in which illness is not only combated, but also interpreted. Where people are not only treated, but also supported. Where you are not just a patient, but a person - in all your fragility, with your questions, your faith, your history. This space does not have to be large. It begins with an honest look, a quiet presence, an open ear. But where it is missing, the illness remains unconnected not only physically, but also emotionally.

5. The desire for encounters and the longing for dignity

At the end of all these experiences is a wish that resonates in almost all stories of seriously ill people: I want to be seen as a human being. This wish is not abstract. It is concrete, physical, psychological. It manifests itself in the desire for a real look, for a touch, for a conversation without time pressure. It manifests itself in the need to be allowed to communicate - without shame, without judgement, without haste.

This longing is also a longing for dignity. Dignity does not mean that everything will be fine - but that someone is there to stay with you when things get difficult. That the self remains, even if the body falls apart. That you don't stop being human just because you have fallen ill. This dignity cannot be prescribed. It can only be given - through attitude, through presence, through the silent promise: You are not alone.

At a time when medicine is becoming ever more precise, technical and efficient, there is a growing danger that this human dimension will be lost. But the more it disappears, the greater the longing for it becomes. And the greater the longing, the greater the pain, if it remains unfulfilled. Indifference is therefore not just a moral problem. It is an attack on what people need most in their vulnerability: proof that they count - not as a case, but as a person.

Chapter 11: When carers fall silent - the silent exhaustion of the helping professions

1. Proximity to suffering as a daily challenge

Nurses are one of the professional groups in the healthcare sector who experience the most intensive and continuous proximity to human suffering. Unlike many medical activities, which take place selectively or episodically, nursing work is characterised by a daily, often hour-long presence at the patient's bedside. It involves not only medical and technical tasks, but also physical care, emotional support and existential presence. This closeness is powerful, touching, meaningful - but at the same time demanding, gruelling and deeply exhausting.

The constant confrontation with pain, deterioration, fear, dying and death requires a high degree of emotional stability. However, in a system that sees care primarily as a resource and not as a relationship, it is precisely these emotional demands that are systematically ignored. Proximity to suffering is not supported, but managed. The compassion that makes this closeness possible is not protected, but assumed. Anyone working in this field of tension needs not only professional expertise, but also inner maturity, emotional resilience and institutional support - all of which are increasingly lacking.

Carers are particularly at risk of falling silent in this situation. Not because they have nothing to say, but because they feel that the system leaves no room for their emotions. Their closeness to the patient, their intuition, their concern often go unheard. Their professionally and humanly sound assessments are ignored, their observations devalued, their excessive demands ignored. What remains is the daily activity - and the feeling that no one sees how much this activity costs.

2. The moral stress between knowing, wanting and not being able to

One of the central psychological burdens of nursing work is what is known as moral stress. This refers to the tension between what one has recognised as right, what one feels is necessary - and what is actually possible in the system. Carers know what would be good: time for a conversation, attentive personal care, empathetic support, appropriate pain therapy. They want to help, alleviate, accompany and comfort. But they are less and less able to do so.

The reason for this does not lie in personal failure, but in the structural conditions: too few staff, too many tasks, too much time pressure, too little recognition, too many hierarchies. This discrepancy between knowing, wanting and not being able to creates a deep feeling of inner turmoil. Many carers develop feelings of guilt, frustration, shame or resignation as a result. They experience themselves as inadequate, even though they surpass themselves every day. This paradoxical constellation - maximum effort with minimum effectiveness - is a breeding ground for quiet despair.

Moral stress is different from physical exhaustion. It goes deeper. It affects self-image, professional identity and inner ethos. And it has a long-term destructive effect if there is no place where it can be expressed, shared and processed. In many organisations, however, precisely this place is missing. There is no regular supervision, no open error culture, no ethical case discussions, no management that listens. So the stress remains unspoken - and continues to have an effect. The result is often indifference: not as a decision, but as petrification.

3. Devaluation, hierarchy and the invisibility of nursing expertise

Nursing is an independent, highly complex and responsible profession. It encompasses medical knowledge, social intelligence, communicative sensitivity, ethical judgement and physical presence. However, in many medical cultures, nursing is not recognised in its entirety. It is seen as "subordinate", "assisting", "performing". Their services are visible - but their expertise often remains invisible. This systemic devaluation has a long history and is deeply rooted in the hierarchical structures of many institutions.

Carers experience time and again that their assessments are not taken seriously. That their observations take second place to medical decisions. That their closeness to patients is not seen as a source of knowledge, but as an emotional speciality. This disregard is not always overt, but it is noticeable: in language, in procedures, in decision-making processes. Those who constantly have to explain themselves, even though they have long since understood, eventually lose the impulse to participate. Those who are not asked stop speaking.

This experience creates a feeling of invisibility. Carers do everything - and yet they are not seen. They do existentially important work - and are marginalised. They bear responsibility - and remain without influence. This discrepancy is not only frustrating. It is degrading. And it has a deep impact on the self-image of those affected. Many withdraw inwardly, speak only the bare minimum, function professionally - but without heart. The indifference is then not an expression of a lack of commitment, but of a deep inner disappointment.

4. The retreat into the functional role as a survival strategy

In a system that does not protect empathy, does not support closeness and does not structurally recognise compassion, carers are often left with only one survival strategy:

retreating into their role. Carers carry out their tasks correctly, efficiently and professionally - but no longer with a personal presence. The function replaces the relationship, the process replaces the attention, the routine replaces the attitude. On the outside, everything seems to work. But internally, much has died.

This withdrawal is often not even conscious. It develops gradually, with every missed break, every overheard hint, every ignored boundary. You don't even realise how you are changing. How your gaze becomes shorter, your voice harsher, your smile rarer. Until one day the thought occurs: "It wasn't like this before." Or: "I don't feel anything anymore." Or: "I can't hold out much longer."

This functional rigidity is dangerous - for the carers themselves and for those who accompany them. Because without resonance, no relationship can develop. And without a relationship, care loses its meaning. But the system does not recognise this loss. It honours performance, not attitude. It measures numbers, not humanity. And so many carers are left in an inner no-man's land: highly resilient, but empty. Professional, but no longer touched. Present, but no longer involved.

5. The silent cry for help: Why indifference is also a sign of pain

When carers appear indifferent, this is rarely an expression of disinterest - but often a silent cry for help. A last chance to protect themselves. An attempt to avoid falling even further. Indifference is then not a moral deficit, but a psychological symptom. It shows that something is missing: resonance, recognition, security, connection. It is the echo of a system that no longer listens. And it is also an appeal - to managers, to colleagues, to society: See us. Hear us. Ask us.

Many carers carry this hardship with them for years. They carry on because they feel responsible. Because they don't want to leave their patients alone. Because they know that their absence would place an even greater burden on others. But inwardly they burn out. And if they then one day resign, fall ill or fall silent, the system is often too late. It registers the failure - but not the cause.

But it would be possible to act differently. With regular dialogue spaces, with a culture of recognition, with good leadership, with genuine participation, with structural support. Above all, however, with an awareness that care is not a mechanical process - but a form of lived humanity. If this humanity is not protected, it will disappear. And with it the dignity of those who try to be there for others every day - with all their strength, with all their closeness, with all their fragility.

Chapter 12: The dangerous power of habituation - How normality breeds indifference

1. The process of blunting through repetition

The psychological mechanics of habituation are based on an evolutionary principle: humans cannot remain permanently in a state of maximum stimulus openness. Repeated stimuli lose intensity - not because they are objectively less significant, but because the nervous system protects itself. This principle can also be seen in medicine, where professional action is accompanied by permanent confrontation with existential issues.

What is still an event of profound emotional impact for the first encounter with death becomes less so with each subsequent case. Not because the event is less significant, but because the reaction to it is weakened by repetition. This psychological necessity poses a double challenge in everyday clinical practice: It enables distance, but jeopardises relationships. It protects the ability to act, but weakens ethical perception. And above all: it imperceptibly changes one's own self-image. A compassionate person becomes a professional subject who seeks refuge in functionality - and over time no longer realises how much they have abandoned themselves.

Repetition therefore not only changes the reaction to the individual event, but also shapes the entire structure of perception. Those who have seen suffering people often enough not only begin to feel less - they also begin to see things differently. What was previously interpreted as an expression of pain now appears as "typical", "predictable", "stressful". The judgement shifts - and with it the willingness to be touched. The individual case becomes a pattern, fate becomes a protocol. Humanity loses weight - not out of indifference, but out of habituation.

2. When the extraordinary becomes commonplace

The medical world is a world of borderline experiences: Birth and death, healing and decay, hope and despair are often only a few metres apart. This density of existential situations represents a constant emotional challenge for those working in it. But the longer you work in this world, the more normal the extraordinary appears. What used to be the exception becomes the rule. What used to take your breath away is becoming the order of the day.

This process is treacherous because it remains invisible. No one consciously chooses to trivialise death and pain. No one chooses to overlook fear and hardship . And yet it happens. A little more every day. Because people adapt - in structures, in language, in behaviour. The exception becomes normality, the normal becomes routine, the empathetic becomes a disruptive factor. And at some point, the signs of suffering are no longer a shock, but a working process.

This reversal has far-reaching consequences for patient care. This is because those affected always experience their situation as exceptional - no matter how often it has already occurred in the system. For the patient, their own diagnosis is a crisis, for the carer it is a standard case. For the relative, imminent death is a life event, for the doctor it is an expected course of events. This asymmetry of perspectives becomes all the more hurtful the less it is recognised. Because it means that what changes everything for me no longer affects you. And it is precisely at this moment that the experience of indifference begins.

3. The creeping shift in moral standards

The change in inner reaction is not only a psychological process, but also a moral one. This is because as we become dull, our conscience also becomes less sensitive. What would previously have triggered an ethical dilemma is now accepted as everyday life. What used to be considered unacceptable is now relativised with a reference to work pressure. The standards are shifting - not through ideology, but through overload, adaptation and repetition.

This shift can go so far that inhumane behaviour is no longer recognised as such. It becomes functionalised, trivialised, professionalised. A patient whose fear is ignored is no longer an ethical problem, but a "difficult case". A dying woman who remains unaccompanied is no longer a catastrophe, but an "organisational gap". Moral language falls silent - replaced by technical, bureaucratic or cynical formulations. Ethical unease is systematically suppressed - and with it the possibility of change.

The person who acts in this way is not evil. He is conformist. They act according to what "works", not according to what is "right". And therein lies the real tragedy of structural indifference: that it is not based on will, but on social conditioning. The shift in standards does not happen because nobody knows what is right any more - but because nobody asks any more.

4. The social protection of the "insensitive"

The normalisation of indifference is not an individual process. It is a social process. In teams, in organisations, in hospital cultures, unspoken rules emerge about how to deal with emotions - or not to deal with them. If you feel too much, you are considered overwhelmed. Those who talk too much are considered exhausting. Those who ask too many questions are considered inefficient. Emotional numbness becomes the norm - not by regulation, but by expectation.

The social reward system is particularly powerful: those who "work" are praised. Those who "stay professional" are encouraged. Those who "work at a distance" are seen as role models. These rewards create behavioural security - and at the same time emotional coldness. Because they signalise: Humanity is not a criterion for success. Closeness is not protected, but sanctioned. Concern is not recognised, but ridiculed.

This culture is not consciously installed - it is created. And that is precisely why it is so powerful. It forms a collective armour that is directed against anything that could disturb it: Tears, sadness, exhaustion, doubt. Anyone who wants to break through this armour needs courage - and often protection from the outside. Because within the system, indifference is not the exception, but the ticket in.

5. Ways back to ethical vigilance in everyday life

But how can we find our way back - from indifference to sensitivity, from routine to responsibility, from numbness to the ethical present? The first step is to recognise the habituation itself. Those who do not realise that they no longer feel anything cannot begin to feel again. It therefore requires a new, conscious perception of one's own inner space: Where am I still touchable? Where do I react - and where do I no longer react? Where has something shifted without me wanting it to?

These questions are uncomfortable - but healing. They re-establish contact with one's own standards. They create space for doubt, for pain, for remorse - but also for change.

The second step is the collective recovery of alertness: through teams that exchange ideas, through leadership that promotes emotional openness, through supervision that interrupts the daily routine. Because moral receptivity is not an individual achievement. It needs resonance.

Above all, however, we need a culture in which ethics, not efficiency, is the measure. In which compassion, not indifference, protects. In which the goal is not normality - but humanity. Only then can familiarisation with suffering once again become what it should be : an opportunity for humility - not for numbness.

Chapter 13: The role of language- When words dehumanise

1. Language as a mirror of inner attitude

Language is always more than just a means of communication - it is an expression of the way we structure, evaluate and inhabit reality. In medicine, this aspect comes into play in a special way, because here we are not just talking about things, but about people in vulnerable, often existential life situations. Anyone who chooses words in this environment is not just choosing concepts - they are establishing, delimiting or dissolving a relationship. Language is therefore not only a mirror of an inner attitude, but also its amplifier, its protective mechanism, its legitimisation.

When a patient is referred to as a "case", this may be useful from an organisational or documentary point of view - but semantically it is a reduction. The "case" has no biography. It has no inner experience, no history, no relatives, no fear. The "case" is an entity within a medical-bureaucratic system, an object of observation, a bearer of values. Such terms relieve those involved because they create distance - but they disenfranchise those affected. They transform subjects into categories, people into tasks.

This form of language is not just individual behaviour, but part of collective routines. Language becomes a social practice that perpetuates a certain understanding of reality: the understanding of the patient as the bearer of a problem that needs to be solved, not as a person who wants to be accompanied. The structure of language shows what counts in the system - and what does not. And anyone who works for a long time with a language in which the subject disappears will at some point see less, feel less and ask fewer questions in their actions.

2. **The loss of personal contact in everyday clinical practice**

A central mechanism of linguistic alienation in the healthcare sector is the loss of direct, personal dialogue. What initially appears to be an organisational necessity - namely communicating about patients with colleagues - becomes the dominant form in everyday life. We talk about people, not with them. The "you" disappears, the "he" and "she" remain. In ward rounds, in meetings, in handovers. Even when the patient is in the room, they are not addressed. They hear what is said about them - but they are not included.

This indirect behaviour is deeply hurtful. It signals: You are not meant. You are there, but you are not part of the conversation. You are described, but not asked. You are being looked at but not spoken to. This phenomenon is particularly dramatic in the case of seriously ill, sedated, demented or dying people, who are often implicitly denied the ability to communicate. Yet it is precisely these people who are particularly dependent on interpersonal presence - also and especially in language.

A personalised approach is not a luxury, but an expression of dignity. It doesn't need time - it needs attention. Anyone who calls a person by name, addresses them directly, greets them, explains what is happening, even if they are supposedly unable to react, is doing something fundamental: You are recognising them. He bears witness to his presence. It gives them the social role of the person being addressed, i.e. a person who is taken seriously. If this role is systematically denied, the result is a double devaluation: physically exposed - and linguistically ignored.

3. Euphemisms, abbreviations and the loss of depth

Another element of linguistic flattening in the medical context is the spread of euphemisms, abbreviations and technocratic terminology. These linguistic strategies arise for pragmatic reasons - they enable efficiency, avoid emotional overload and ensure communicative control. But they have side effects. They reduce complex, often deeply human experiences to functional terms that no longer allow any inner movement.

If, for example, the term "ex" is used instead of "deceased person", then the event of death disappears from the linguistic space. If we talk about "providing food" instead of "eating together", then an interpersonal situation becomes a logistical process. When the word "levelling out" describes the dying process, life itself becomes a dosage. The linguistic approach not only changes the description, but also the experience of reality - it becomes smoother, more predictable, more distanced.

These terms are not wrong, but they are incomplete. They are technically correct, but existentially hollow. They name processes, but they conceal what these processes mean. And therein lies their risk: they relieve those involved of the need to localise themselves emotionally and morally. You no longer have to mourn when someone "exists". You no longer have to sympathise when someone is "derailed". Language becomes armour, sedation, a moral shield - and thus also a source of silent indifference.

4. Linguistic distance as a form of professional self-relief

However, these linguistic strategies are not merely an expression of a lack of attitude, but often an act of self-care. Those who are confronted with severe suffering on a daily basis develop linguistic means of distancing themselves. This distance is initially helpful - it creates clarity, enables efficiency and maintains the ability to act. But when it becomes a permanent attitude, it loses its relieving function and becomes the norm. Then language no longer protects against excessive demands - it prevents connection.

Professional communication is often portrayed in training as factual, emotion-free and clearly defined. This idea characterises the self-image of many young professionals. They learn that compassion is not intended in language. That emotions should be replaced by neutral wording. That a "difficult conversation" is less difficult if you find the right words - words that calm, soften, depersonalise. But this begins a gradual process: language loses its access to the inner truth. And with it, the ego also loses its connection to itself.

In such a linguistic environment, it becomes increasingly difficult to be authentic. Anyone who senses that compassion cannot find linguistic expression suppresses it. Those who realise that doubts cannot be expressed remain silent. And anyone who experiences that language only works will eventually lose the ability to use it to connect with others. What remains is a professional role - but no longer a linguistic space for humanity.

5. Ways to humanise language in a medical context

Human medicine needs a language that not only names, but also touches. A language that not only controls, but also allows. A language that not only informs, but also enters into a relationship. The first step towards this lies in raising awareness: What terms do we use every day - and what do they do to us? Which language habits protect us - and which ones separate us from what we actually feel?

This awareness can be promoted through reflection processes in teams, language-sensitive training, regular collegial case discussions and a management culture of openness. It can be supported by supervision sessions in which not only content but also forms of expression are discussed. It can be strengthened by a culture in which language is understood as part of the relationship - not just as a means to an end.

Above all, however, the spoken word needs to be rehabilitated as an ethical act. Anyone who calls a dying person by name in their presence recognises them. Anyone who tells a relative the truth - clearly but compassionately - heals. Those who allow their own insecurities to be spoken in a team free others from the burden of pretence. Such language is not perfect. It is often tentative, fragile, imperfect. But it is genuine. And its power lies in its authenticity.

Because when words mean people again, compassion can return. Where language creates relationships again, healing begins - not only in the body, but also between people. And where this happens, indifference no longer has a place. Not because it has been banished - but because it has become superfluous.

Chapter 14: Lack of ethics as a system error- when moral orientation is lost

1. Medicine as an ethically charged practice

Medical action is never purely technical, never neutral, never purely functional. It is inevitably caught between life and death, between helping and intervening, between responsibility and powerlessness. Every decision in medicine - whether diagnostic, therapeutic, organisational or communicative - has an ethical dimension. For it concerns not only bodies, but people; not only processes, but destinies; not only symptoms, but contexts of meaning.

This basic ethical tension is not an add-on, not a luxury, not a moral decoration. It is part of the essence of medicine. It is reflected in the question of how to deal with uncertainty, how to set priorities, how to deal with limited resources, how to speak to the dying, how to weigh up medical feasibility and human reasonableness. Medical decisions are never just right or wrong - they are always good or bad in a moral sense. And this is precisely why medicine needs a reliable, present, lived ethical orientation.

However, in many areas of the modern healthcare system, this orientation seems to have been lost . Although ethics are discussed, taught and formulated in guiding principles, they are rarely reflected in everyday life. It is institutionally present, but not culturally anchored. It is available as a concept, but not tangible as an attitude. And it is precisely in this gap - between knowledge and reality - that a dangerous vacuum is created: a system that is technically highly competent but morally directionless.

2. The invisibility of ethical issues in everyday clinical practice

One of the main problems of modern medicine is that ethical issues are often no longer recognised as such. They disappear under time pressure, process optimisation, standardisation and bureaucratisation. Decisions that have a profound impact on a person's life - such as whether a therapy should be started, continued or ended, whether an intervention is still indicated or whether resuscitation should be avoided - are often made on purely medical or organisational grounds. The ethical dimension is suppressed, overlooked and devalued.

This invisibility is all the more dangerous because it is subtle. Nobody decides to be ethically blind. It simply happens - because there is no time, because there is no space, because there is no culture in which such issues can be discussed. The focus is on feasibility, on safety, on speed - not on meaning, on relationships, on humanity. As a result, even serious decisions end up in a grey area in which they are formally correct but inwardly hollow.

The result is a clinical everyday life in which action is possible without any moral constraints. Therapies are carried out because they are available - not because they make sense. People are sedated because it is easier - not because it is right in the individual case. Relatives are put off because it creates less conflict - not because it is respectful. And above all of this lies a basic feeling: that you just work, that there is no other way, that you have no choice. But this is precisely the symptom of a lost ethical orientation.

3. Economisation, hierarchy and ethical speechlessness

A central reason for the disappearance of ethical reflection lies in the increasing economisation of the healthcare system. Hospitals are run as businesses, medical activities are evaluated in economic terms and decisions are controlled by business management. Under these conditions, ethics is often perceived as a disruptive factor - as an obstacle to efficiency, as a brake on throughput times, as a burden on flat rates per case. It is either marginalised or instrumentalised - but rarely taken seriously.

Added to this is the hierarchical structure of many medical institutions. In a culture in which decisions are made top-down and dissent is seen as disloyalty, ethical reflection is hardly possible. This is because it thrives on open dialogue, on weighing things up, on jointly searching for the right in the wrong. However, if critical voices are not heard, uncertainties are not shared and questions are not allowed to be asked, then ethics falls silent - not because it is missing, but because there is no longer any room for it.

This structural speechlessness leads to a fatal dynamic: anyone who expresses doubts is considered inefficient. Anyone who argues morally is considered naive. Anyone who questions decisions is considered uncomfortable. This creates an atmosphere of conformity in which not only action but also thought becomes indifferent. People do what is expected - and no longer question whether it is good. Getting used to the morally questionable becomes part of the professional identity. And with every unasked question, ethics becomes a bit more of a blind spot.

4. Ethics as individual responsibility or collective practice?

Another reason for the disappearance of lived ethics lies in the misunderstanding of their localisation. In many medical contexts, ethics is seen as a personal attitude: those who act morally do so out of their own conviction. However, this individualisation overburdens the individual and relieves the system. This is because it shifts responsibility to areas where it cannot be borne alone - and leaves a void where it would be institutionally necessary.

Ethics is not a private matter. It is a collective practice. It needs places where it can take place: in teams, in case discussions, in supervision, in training courses. It needs people who make it possible: through leadership, through attitude, through listening. And it needs structures that protect it: Time, protection, methods, openness. Only then can an ethical culture emerge from moral intuition - a culture that not only aims to make the right decision, but also to struggle for it together.

This also includes admitting that there is often no clear-cut solution. That ethics does not mean knowing everything - but being prepared to ask questions. That it does not primarily want to do the right thing - but to do it responsibly. Such ethics are not weak, but strong. Not disruptive, but stabilising. And it doesn't start with the big discourse, but with the small question: Is it allowed to be like this?

5. Steps towards the ethical re-centring of medical practice

If indifference is an expression of repressed or absent ethics, then the key to change lies in reclaiming them. The ethical re-centring of medical action does not mean installing another set of rules. It means creating spaces in which questions are allowed again. In which uncertainty is not seen as a weakness, but as a sign of depth. Where it is not about fulfilling norms, but about shared responsibility.

A first step is to revitalise ethical case discussions - not as an exception, but as a routine. Situations in which people suffer, die or despair must be discussed - not just professionally, but morally. Formats are needed in which the question is asked: Did we act correctly? What moved us? What did we miss? What did we need? This is the only way to create a space in which attitudes can grow.

A second step is the integration of ethics into training. Not as a module, but as an attitude. Not as theory, but as practice. Medical professions must learn that decisions are never purely technical - they are always an expression of a world view, an appreciation of the human being, a relationship to life. This reflection must be part of professionalisation from the outset - otherwise it will remain alien later on.

A third step lies in institutional support. Ethics officers, clinical ethics committees and ethical guidelines are important instruments - but they are not enough. The decisive question is: Are ethics practised? Is it being asked? Is it wanted? And is it protected? Where this happens, medical practice can once again become what it originally was: an art of helping, a form of assistance, a place of responsibility. And that is precisely the opposite of indifference.

Chapter 15: When the system makes you ill - burnout, depression and moral exhaustion in the healthcare system

1. The healthcare system as a high-risk environment for mental exhaustion

In hardly any other professional field is the density of existential challenges as great as in medicine. The daily confrontation with suffering, death, chronic illness, social hardship, ethical dilemmas and emotional powerlessness requires a permanent emotional responsiveness - while at the same time being functionally available at all times. This double burden, combined with a chronic lack of resources, recognition and emotional feedback, represents a psychological high-risk profile. Added to this is the fact that medical staff are socialised to suppress their own needs: to function even when it hurts, to remain present even when you are exhausted inside, to appear strong even though you feel weak.

This constellation is not accidental. It is the result of a system that is designed for continuous performance, but not for psychological integrity. There are hardly any institutionalised spaces for emotionality, hardly any structurally secured opportunities for self-care, hardly any protected forms of dealing with exhaustion. Those who can no longer cope are considered overwhelmed - not the system. Those who remain silent protect themselves - but reinforce the cultural logic of denial. This creates an atmosphere in which systemically induced exhaustion is not only not addressed, but is often even reinterpreted as a measure of professionalism.

2. Burnout as a collapse between commitment and reality

The typical course of a burnout does not begin with indifference, but with idealism. People who are involved in helping professions are highly motivated, responsible and meaningful. They go above and beyond without realising it at first - because the drive comes not from pressure, but from conviction. But this is precisely where the danger lies: if the commitment is not reciprocated, if feedback is lacking, if organisational or economic limits prevent any form of genuine relationship, a slow erosion of inner meaning begins.

In advanced burnout, doing loses its meaning. The former enthusiasm turns into emotional numbness, the desire to help gives way to the urge to survive. Relationships with patients are functionalised, emotional reactions are flattened, compassion is suppressed. The professional mask remains - but it has become hollow. The subject has withdrawn from their own actions. This inner separation is not intentional, it is suffered - a psychological self-protection that becomes a condition.

Burnout cannot be equated with mere exhaustion. It is not a temporary low mood, but a comprehensive loss of emotional coherence. The person affected does not recognise themselves and perceives their own behaviour as alien, distant and empty. The danger of indifference lies precisely in this inner alienation: it is not intentional, but a consequence of the feeling that you can no longer give anything because you have already lost everything inside.

3. Moral exhaustion- when acting against your own convictions makes you ill

In contrast to burnout, which refers to overload due to quantity, moral exhaustion describes the suffering from a contradiction between one's own ethos and the external framework for action. This condition is particularly common in nursing, but also among doctors, therapists, social workers and counsellors. Those affected not only feel exhausted - they feel torn inside. They want to help - and are not allowed to . They know what would be right - and have to do the opposite.

These moral dilemmas arise, for example, when unnecessary treatments are carried out because there is economic pressure. When patients die without adequate care because there is a lack of staff. When there is no time for dialogue, even though it is urgently needed. When documentation is more important than human contact. In such situations, a slow process of internal erosion begins. Moral integrity is not directly violated - it is eroded by the system on a daily basis. And at some point you start to doubt: not only the system, but also yourself.

The symptoms of moral exhaustion often resemble depression or burnout in their outward appearance, but their core is different: it is not fatigue, but inner guilt that cannot be articulated. It is the awareness of being involved in the suffering of others, even though you wanted the opposite. This guilt is often difficult to name because it is not based on specific misbehaviour, but on systemic complicity. And it is precisely this lack of clarity that makes it so destructive.

4. Depression as an expression of silent despair in the system

If burnout and moral exhaustion go unnoticed or untreated for a long time, they can lead to depressive states. However, depression in a medical context often has a specific face: it is not a retreat to bed, but rather a shutdown on duty. It is not the failure of the task, but the mechanical continuation of functioning without inner involvement. The person affected laughs, documents, advises - but no longer feels anything. They are not absent - but they are no longer there either.

This form of functional depression is particularly difficult to recognise because it fits perfectly into the logic of the system. It does not disturb, it does not rebel, it does not question. It fulfils its duty, but it no longer has an inner place. People have become invisible in their own profession - not to others, but to themselves. The self-image collapses, one's own actions appear hollow, the connection to other people evaporates. In this silence lies the deepest form of medical indifference: indifference to oneself.

Such conditions can lead to serious psychosomatic consequences, chronic exhaustion and suicidal tendencies - not from a sudden impulse, but from continued inner emptying. If the system offers no places where this emptiness can be talked about, it becomes the norm. And it is precisely in this normality that the system's deepest illness lies: it does not recognise its exhausted people - because it is exhausted itself.

5. From symptom to change- an appeal to the system

As long as mental exhaustion is treated as an individual problem, its systemic cause remains untouched. Resilience training, mindfulness courses and work-life balance programmes are important - but they fall short. This is because they suggest that those affected have to adapt to a sick system instead of the system being committed to the humanity of its members. Real change begins where structures are created that not only enable care, but demand it.

These structures must be more than therapeutic interventions. They must create cultural conditions in which compassion becomes a competence rather than a danger. This includes a new definition of leadership that not only guides, but protects. A new practice of supervision that not only controls, but accompanies. A new language about exhaustion that relieves rather than shames. And a new form of collegiality that is not based on performance, but on humanity.

We need a system that doesn't lose its people. One that doesn't ask: "How much can you still give?" but rather: "Will you still be seen?" A system that does not function at the expense of those who support it. Rather, one that begins with its care - with those who help others. Because indifference doesn't just arise from excessive demands. It arises from a lack of reflection, of reconnection, of encounter. And those who allow people in the system to meet again - themselves, each other, the patients - begin to heal it.

6. Structural prevention- How systems can remain human

If mental exhaustion, moral withdrawal and emotional numbness are understood not as individual failures but as an expression of systemic overload, then prevention requires a structural response. It is not the individual who must adapt to an illness-causing system - the system itself must be designed in such a way that humanity, compassion and reflection can survive within it. Such structural prevention is not an "add-on", not an additional offer for exceptional cases, but a central element of organisational responsibility and a culture of care.

Structural prevention begins with what is visible and permitted in the organisational culture. In a functioning system, it is possible - even desirable - to talk openly about emotional stress, inner doubts and ethical tensions. This requires spaces in which medical professionals can meet each other beyond the pressure of efficiency and hierarchy: Supervisions, ethical case discussions, collegial counselling, interprofessional reflection groups. Such formats must not depend on the goodwill of individuals or remain optional in their implementation - they must be a mandatory, structured and institutionally secured part of everyday working life.

A second key element is a management culture that not only manages performance, but also shares responsibility for mental well-being. Managers must be able to recognise emotional exhaustion, recognise signs of withdrawal or cynicism and offer support at an early stage. This requires a new type of management training that recognises psychosocial competence not as a soft skill, but as a core qualification. A manager who categorises exhaustion as weakness or unprofessionalism is reproducing the system that should actually be protecting them.

A third preventative element is the structural anchoring of time - not just for tasks, but for relationships. In many institutions, there is systematically too little time for direct communication, for real presence, for processing and interpersonal relationships. Appointments, ward rounds and case discussions are tightly scheduled, breaks are shortened and personal conversations are squeezed into free time. A system that deals with time in this way forces alienation. It prevents compassion, not because it wants to - but because it leaves no room for it. Structural prevention therefore also means recognising time as a basic human need - not as an economic residual.

A fourth building block is the establishment of transparent, psychologically sound protective mechanisms against chronic overwork. These include working time models with real recovery phases, rotation systems for particularly stressful stations, a fair distribution of tasks, stress-sensitive duty rosters and the right to temporary relief in the event of inner exhaustion - without this being linked to a loss of career or feelings of guilt. Catching people before they break not only prevents mental illness, but also preserves the quality of medical relationships.

There is also a need for a language that does not taboo psychological experiences. In many medical systems, exhaustion is not talked about - for fear of stigmatisation, loss of face, rejection. Structural prevention means breaking through this speechlessness. Internal communication strategies are needed in where mental well-being is seen as part of professional integrity - not as a private problem. Managers need to be able to talk about their own exhaustion without losing authority. And it needs teams that not only tolerate openness, but support it.

Ultimately, however, structural prevention begins with a change of perspective: from the idea of "functioning personnel" to the reality of "vulnerable people with responsibility". Those who recognise the fragility of medical professions not as a risk, but as an anthropological fact, will begin to build systems that can deal with this truth. And only when the system itself becomes human can it demand that its members maintain humanity. Anything else is excessive demands - and thus: Indifference as a reaction.

Chapter 16: The great silence- Why indifference is not talked about

1. Indifference as a blind spot of the institution

In medical facilities, there are countless indicators for performance, efficiency, hygiene, cost-effectiveness and quality - but hardly any for humanity. There are sophisticated systems for measuring waiting times, case numbers, length of stay and treatment costs, but no reliable structures for recording interpersonal presence, ethical behaviour or emotional resonance. The result is an institutional blindness to what is at the centre of human encounters: empathic presence.

This blindness is not accidental. It has grown structurally. It has become established because it protects the system - from excessive demands, from ethical conflict, from complexity. Because anyone who takes indifference seriously would have to scrutinise how it arises. They would have to ask why nobody stops. They would have to examine whether what works is also good. Instead, the issue is suppressed - not out of malice, but out of habit. And so indifference itself becomes part of the system: invisible, but effective. Unrecognised, but present.

This invisibility has fatal consequences. Because what is not named cannot be dealt with. What is not expressed remains effective - as a shadow, as a mood, as silent poison. Those who work in an environment in which indifference is not allowed to be discussed begin to believe that it is normal. And those who no longer recognise it become part of its transmission - not because they want to, but because they can no longer do otherwise.

2. Fear of your own sensitivity

A central reason for remaining silent about indifference lies in the fear of what would become apparent if it were named. Those who talk about indifference also talk about their own experiences: about the moments when they didn't listen, didn't react, didn't ask. About the guilty conscience that was pushed aside in the hustle and bustle of everyday life. About the compassion that you lost at some point. About the pain that was too great to admit. Silence is therefore a form of self-protection - against guilt, against shame, against being overwhelmed.

This defence is understandable. After all, indifference is not just behaviour - it is a state that arises in us when something can no longer be felt. Anyone who notices it has to confront their own numbness. With the question: When did I stop being touched? When did I start to just function? When did I become indifferent to the suffering of others ? These questions touch on deep, often painful layers of the professional self-image - and that is precisely why they are often not asked.

What's more: In an environment where emotional strength is equated with professional competence, there is an implicit stigma attached to admitting a loss of empathy. Anyone who says that nothing touches them anymore fears that they are no longer suitable. Anyone who admits that they are becoming numb is questioning themselves. In this culture of inner defence, silence becomes a condition for carrying on. But this silence comes at a price: it makes the unsaid permanently effective.

3. The normalisation of the deviant

A particularly perfidious mechanism for dealing with indifference is its normalisation. What used to be considered unacceptable - such as leaving a room without saying a word, ignoring emotional distress, devaluing patients during handover - is taken for granted in many teams. It's "just the way it is", "part of the job", "everyone does it". This normalisation is not only a defence, but also a systemic legitimisation. The deviation becomes the standard. The exception becomes the rule. Indifference becomes the norm.

This development is stabilised by the linguistic and social routines in the team. Anyone who asks whether the behaviour was appropriate is considered sensitive. Anyone who criticises the fact that a patient has been overlooked disrupts the process. Anyone who points out interpersonal deficits is ridiculed or ignored. This indifference is not only tolerated - it is socially protected. And those who avoid it often find themselves alone.

In this culture of collective silence, the newcomers also begin to adapt. Young colleagues who are still highly sensitive quickly realise that their compassion is seen as naïve, their commitment as excessive and their reflection as time-consuming. They learn that those who want to belong remain silent. Those who want to belong look the other way. Those who want to belong, work. This is how indifference is reproduced - not by regulation, but by socialisation.

4. The myth of professional distance

Another reason for the silence about indifference lies in a widespread misunderstanding: the myth of professional distance. In many training contexts, it is suggested that medical action is only professional if it remains emotion-free. Closeness is associated with danger, empathy with excessive demands, compassion with instability. The result is a culture of internal compartmentalisation: the person in the white coat is allowed to see everything - but feel nothing. May decide everything - but question nothing. Allowed to do everything - but not to doubt.

This myth prevents the thematisation of indifference. Because as long as emotional detachment is considered a necessary competence, any criticism of coldness or apathy appears to be a misunderstanding. You have to remain "professional", they say. You shouldn't get "too involved". And so indifference is not categorised as a shortcoming, but as a sign of maturity. Those who are affected are "not in control". Those who are not affected are "in control". But this reinterpretation is dangerous. Because it confuses emotional absence with control - and compassion with weakness.

Professional distance does not mean feeling nothing. It means remaining receptive - and at the same time able to act. It means not losing yourself - but not closing yourself off either. And this is precisely the challenge: maintaining compassion without breaking. Those who instead declare indifference to be the norm are not protecting the subject - they are slowly killing their moral resilience.

5. Ways out of silence- the return to language

The first step out of silence is to find language again. If you want to talk about indifference, you need words, spaces and relationships in which it is possible to speak. It needs formulations that describe rather than accuse. It needs a tone that does not moralise, but opens up. And it needs a counterpart who does not listen, but goes along.

This language cannot be prescribed. It must be developed, tested and protected together. It begins in small gestures: in asking about the experience of a situation, in talking after a stressful shift, in pausing after a death. It begins with the willingness to name what you feel again - even if it is uncomfortable. And it begins with the decision that humanity is not an add-on - but the core of professionalism.

When indifference is talked about again, more than just a process of realisation takes place. A new space is created: a space of relationship, of responsibility, of transformation. In this space, people can once again feel what moves them. They can see again what they have lost. They can recognise again that indifference is not guilt - but a call. A call to not give up on yourself. And it is precisely this call that begins where silence ends.

Chapter 17: Silent connivance- How indifference becomes entrenched in teams

1. The individual in the collective- How moral impulses get lost

The first experience of many newcomers to the medical profession is not professional overload, but moral irritation. The first night watch, the first death of a patient, the first conversation with desperate relatives - all these experiences challenge an ethos that is usually idealistic, touchable and openly carried into the profession. But it soon becomes clear that asking too many questions, feeling too much and pausing too long disrupts the work. And so moral impulses come into contradiction with practice: they come up against routines, disinterest, speechless processes.

Within teams, this contradiction is often not dealt with, but resolved through self-adjustment. Individuals begin to no longer take their irritation seriously, to relativise their own feelings, to interpret their own sensitivity as weakness. This does not happen out of indifference - but out of a deep need for connection, for belonging, for protection. The group becomes the norm - and anything that deviates from it appears suspicious. Moral impulses are lost - not because they disappear, but because they find no support.

This dynamic is dangerous because it turns conscience into a private problem. Ethical perception is decoupled from collective practice. What is felt internally must not appear externally. And so the system begins to silence the very people who should be supporting it - the empathetic, the doubters, the questioners - in its practice.

2. Group norms and the principle of unspoken consensus

Teams operate not only according to rosters and instructions, but above all according to invisible rules: Who is allowed to say what? What can be thought? When is behaviour unacceptable - and when is it tacitly accepted? These group norms are created through repetition, implicit rewards and informal sanctions. If you conform to them, you belong. Those who break them are quickly marginalised.

The principle of unspoken consensus acts like a collective cloak of invisibility here. Everyone knows that there are situations in which patients are not seen, needs are ignored, statements are dismissed. And yet we don't talk about it - not out of ignorance, but because no-one is leading the way. The unspoken consensus is: we do what is necessary. We don't ask what would be right . We get on with it. And this "we" protects the individual - and ties them down at the same time.

This consensus stabilises particularly where hierarchies are not made permeable through open communication. In rigid structures, there is no reflection, but rather expectation. Senior physicians set the tone, ward managers define what is normal. And so a culture develops in which moral thinking is not acted out, but subordinated. In this context, indifference does not appear to be a disruption - but a necessary attitude to safeguard operations.

3. Loyalty as a moral dilemma

Loyalty is highly valued in many clinical teams - and with good reason. Those who work with others under pressure, bear responsibility on night duty and overcome crises together develop a deep collegial bond. This solidarity is supportive, but also dangerous. Because it interweaves moral judgement with emotional affiliation. Criticising a colleague becomes a breach of loyalty. Pointing out a colleague's indifference becomes a breach of trust. Moral judgement is personalised - not objectively, but socially weighted.

In this constellation, every ethical statement is also a risk: for the climate, for the relationship, for one's own standing. Anyone who speaks out must reckon with exclusion - or subtle isolation. More often, however, the opposite happens: you don't speak. The silent look, the ironic remark, the private complaint are all that remain. The moral conflict is not resolved - it is externalised. The blame is delegated: to the system, to the overload, to the circumstances. And so loyalty becomes a substitute for ethical self-responsibility.

This dynamic can only be overcome through conscious separation: Collegiality must not be confused with complicity. Closeness must not be understood as protection from criticism. And cohesion must not be based on silence about the unspeakable. A mature team culture recognises that loyalty is not created through concealment, but through honesty - even where it hurts.

4. The dynamics of collective displacement

The longer indifference remains unthematised in a team, the more deeply anchored the collective repression becomes. Routines of not feeling arise: joking dressing-up, cynical comments, functionalised language, ritualised moving on. What initially serves as psychological relief becomes a professional attitude. The emotional distress is not only hidden - at some point it appears inappropriate.

This dynamic is particularly difficult to break through because it does not react to arguments. It thrives on atmosphere, hints and glances. Anyone who enters the room and senses that an incident is not to be talked about will silently conform. Anyone who realises that grief is seen as weakness will not grieve. And anyone who realises that touching has become taboo will no longer allow themselves to be touched. Emotional reality is replaced - by adaptation.

The fatal thing about this collective repression is that it binds the team internally. On the outside, it appears stable, efficient and loyal. But on the inside, there is an emotional void, ethical insecurity and psychological exhaustion. No one is alone - and yet everyone is thrown back on themselves. In this silence, indifference grows - not as a decision, but as a result of systematic self-denial.

5. Ways out of the silent complicity

The return from collective repression begins with a gesture: the gesture of seeing again. It happens in a sentence that does not judge, but describes. In a question that does not lament, but connects. In a moment in which someone says: "I realise that this no longer touches me - and that scares me." Such sentences can open up spaces in which others join in - not out of obligation, but out of relief.

Institutional permission is needed for such spaces to emerge: supervision sessions in which not only professional but also human dialogue takes place. Case discussions in which the unspoken also has a place. Ethics discussions in which the right thing is not prescribed, but sought together. But it also requires the courage of the individual - the courage to leave the protection of silence. Not to be better than the others, but to make what we have in common possible again.

Because indifference is not the opposite of caring - it is its negative inverse. It indicates where something that was once there has been lost. And it can disappear when what we have in common is renewed - not through regulations, but through relationships. A team that once again feels that it is jointly responsible will begin to listen anew. And this listening is the first step towards healing - not only of the patients, but also of themselves.

Chapter 18: The return of compassion - What helps against indifference

1. Compassion as a reconstructive force in the face of the systemic

Compassion is more than a spontaneous emotional impulse - it is an ethically structured capacity for inner resonance. It means tuning into the suffering of another without sinking into it. It encompasses perception, judgement and a tendency to act - in other words, a complex interplay of cognitive, affective and motivational processes. Compassion is therefore not a naïve or sentimental gesture, but a highly differentiated expression of human connection - and a psychologically stable counterweight to alienation, objectification and functional coldness.

In a system that is designed for efficiency, reproducibility and distance, compassion initially acts as a disruptive factor. It delays processes, questions decisions, makes circumstances visible that the system prefers to ignore. But its systemic function lies precisely in this disruption: it reminds us of what has been forgotten through routine. It prevents the system from functioning solely as a machine. It is a marker for human vitality - not despite, but because of its irritating power.

Compassion is therefore not only an inner resource, but also a corrective. It indicates where something is missing, where something is happening too quickly, where a person is disappearing. If it is given space in everyday medical practice, it acts like an early warning system - not loudly, but unmistakably. And if it is permanently suppressed, this does not show the maturity of the institution, but rather its incipient moral degeneration.

2. The neurobiology of resonance - compassion as a natural disposition

From a neurobiological perspective, compassion is not an exceptional moral achievement, but is deeply rooted in the human organism. At the latest with the discovery of mirror neurons, it became clear that we react to the experience of others not only out of social learning, but also from a basic biological structure. Humans are capable of co-resonance - not as a luxury, but as a condition of their social existence. This means that even in a medical context, compassion is there to begin with - it does not have to be generated, but rather protected from being superimposed.

Stress, time pressure, hierarchy, excessive demands and cynicism act neurobiologically as blockades of these resonance systems. They partially switch off the prefrontal cortex - the instance for social regulation - but activate the autonomous stress centres. The result is a state of functional self-defence: The other person is no longer perceived as a fellow human being, but as a task, problem or burden.

Compassion has not disappeared - it is neurophysiologically blocked. And this is precisely why it can be reactivated through structural relief.

This leads to a key realisation: compassion can be trained, nurtured and supported. It is not an either-or, but a dynamic process. And this process can be influenced - through language, attitude, relationships, but also through framework conditions. Giving space reduces the release of cortisol. Speaking activates social networks in the brain. Those who are touched open up internally. All of this shows that indifference is not a basic state - it is a reaction to excessive demands. And compassion is not a weakness - but a sign of inner openness.

3. The ethics of small steps - compassion as a means of action

One of the most important mistakes in dealing with indifference is the idea that it can only be dealt with through major reforms. But compassion cannot be decreed - it has to emerge. It does not begin in committees, but in moments. In a decision not to move on immediately. In a gaze that does not flinch. In a gesture that does not break off. The return of compassion happens in everyday life - not at the level of theory, but in concrete action.

This ethic of small steps is radical in its modesty. It makes no claim to improving the world - but it quietly resists brutalisation. It does not ask: "What can I do?", but: "Where can I be human now?" This question is subversive - because it undermines the system without fighting it. It is relieving - because it opens up room for manoeuvre where previously there was only powerlessness. And it is unifying - because it creates a relationship where previously there was isolation.

Compassion often shows itself where no one expects it. In the tired voice that still listens. In the exhausted hand that still holds. In the full day when a quiet conversation still takes place. These gestures are not efficient - but they have an effect. They leave their mark on others - and on our own conscience. And that is precisely why they are indispensable: they write a different narrative into everyday life. A narrative of touch - against the great silence.

4. Collective empathy- when systems become healing

Compassion can also be a collective quality. Teams, wards, clinics, entire institutions can develop an atmosphere in which compassion is not only allowed, but desired. Such atmospheres are not the result of happy accidents - they are created through conscious work on language, rituals, communication and leadership. They thrive on role models who show themselves without losing themselves. From colleagues who ask questions instead of condemning. From superiors who listen, even when there is nothing to "solve".

In such systems, compassion is not treated as an individual risk, but as a collective value. It is protected - through a culture of open dialogue, through time windows for reflection, through supervision, through a culture of breaks. It is encouraged - through further training, feedback and ethical case discussions. And it is rewarded - not with bonuses, but with meaning.

This collective capacity for compassion is not an ideal, but an achievable reality. It requires systems to ask themselves what they are there for: For patients or for process figures? For encounters or for documentation? For performance or for meaning? The answer does not lie in exclusivity - but in balance. And this balance begins where people meet again as people - in their vulnerability, in their limitations, in their longing for meaning.

5. Reconnecting with the origin

Compassion is the origin of medical practice. Not the knowledge of medicines, not the mastery of equipment, not the mastery of procedures - but the ability to be touched by the suffering of another is the reason why people enter this profession. Indifference arises when this origin is lost. And it disappears when it is found again.

This reconnection does not require new training, additional resources or external changes. It needs memories: of the first moment when you wanted to help. The first time you were touched. The face of a patient who stayed. A conversation that was more than routine. In these memories lies the power to remember why you do what you do. And from this memory grows a new present.

So compassion is not just a reaction - it is a return. A return to our own history. A return to meaning. A return to humanity. And this is precisely where its deepest power lies: it not only heals others - it also heals ourselves.

Chapter 19: Between aspiration and reality- Why humanity is not a sure-fire success

1. The myth of the good- between vocation and excessive demands

The medical profession is traditionally understood not only as an activity, but also as a vocation - an inner ethos that is committed to helping, serving and giving of oneself. This myth of the good pervades biographical narratives, letters of motivation, training programmes and institutional models. It provides meaning, stability and a high level of moral identification. At the same time, however, it creates a pressure of expectation that hardly anyone can withstand in the long term.

This is because the ethos of vocation goes hand in hand with the unspoken idea that humanity is self-evident - that it realises itself through good will. But this is precisely a misconception. Humanity is not an automatic consequence of values, but a daily challenge - fragile, contingent, contradictory. Those who treat it as a matter of course ignore its conditionality. And those who see it as a moral duty risk overburdening themselves. The myth of vocation ignores the fact that people are vulnerable in the system - that they have limited resources, that they can fail, that they also need to be protected.

In this tension between ideal and reality, an inner conflict often develops that is invisible but effective: the moral standards are high - but they leave no room for deviation. Those who measure up to them must experience themselves as inadequate. Those who fail are to blame. Those who feel too little have lost themselves. In this way, high standards turn into silent self-judgement - and the desire to help turns into a retreat into functioning. In this movement, humanity not only loses its depth, but also its authenticity.

2. The institutional staging of humanity- façade or substance?

Humanity is omnipresent in the external communication of medical facilities: patients are portrayed as partners, empathy as a leitmotif, individualised care as a matter of course. These narratives are effective - not only externally, but also internally. They define what is desired as a guiding principle. But if they stand in sharp contrast to the reality experienced, they lose their uplifting power. They become a façade.

This façade has a paradoxical effect: it protects the system - but it discourages people. Because anyone who experiences on a daily basis that closeness is impossible in terms of time, individual care is organisationally undesirable or personal attention is structurally hindered, experiences the discrepancy between image and reality as a devaluation of their own perception. The ideal remains - but it becomes irredeemable. The result is a creeping disillusionment: those who permanently live against their own ideal begin to question it. Or worse still - they stop feeling it.

In this situation, the system begins to immunise itself. Criticism of the gap between aspiration and reality is devalued as a lack of resilience. Sadness over lost relationships is interpreted as weakness. The desire for more humanity is dismissed as unrealistic nostalgia. This creates a climate of moral rigidity: ideals remain sacrosanct - but they can no longer be seriously demanded. Humanity becomes a rhetorical shell - and in this shell, indifference remains invisible.

3. The psychodynamic price of the functional self

The gap between aspiration and reality in the medical profession is not only an institutional problem, but also a psychodynamic one. Those who constantly act in a role that they can no longer fulfil inwardly split themselves off - consciously or unconsciously - from their feelings. This splitting off is a protective mechanism: it prevents the self from being torn apart by its inner discrepancy. But it has a price. It creates emptiness.

This emptiness is not immediately noticeable. It manifests itself in a loss of inner resonance, in a functional self that fulfils all requirements - but no longer feels. People in this state no longer really meet other people. They fulfil tasks, follow standards, communicate diagnoses - but they are inwardly absent. The indifference is not intentional - it is suffered. And it is not always visible - but it characterises the atmosphere.

The psychodynamic consequence is deep insecurity: those who no longer feel themselves begin to doubt their own profession. Those who have become alienated from their own compassion ask themselves whether they are still a good doctor or a good carer at all. But because the admission of this alienation is associated with guilt, shame and weakness, it remains unspoken. An inner vacuum is created - a space in which indifference becomes the new normal, unnoticed.

4. The ethical erosion caused by structural violence

Structural violence is a term from the social sciences that describes how social systems harm people without this violence being visible or attributable to specific individuals. In the medical context, this means that if a system permanently maintains conditions that prevent humanity, make closeness difficult, devalue relationships and prevent reflection, a climate of moral erosion is created - without anyone being explicitly responsible.

This form of violence works quietly, indirectly, but constantly. It manifests itself in overcrowded duty rosters, in time pressure, in a lack of supervision, in silent teams, in the prioritisation of economic over human interests. And it has a double effect: it not only damages patient care - it also damages the moral integrity of those providing care. Because it forces them to act against their own conscience, to suppress closeness, to ignore boundaries.

This experience leaves its mark. Those who are repeatedly rendered morally powerless lose faith in their own ethical self-efficacy. Those who regularly have to act against what they inwardly believe to be right not only become numb - their moral identity breaks down. And this is precisely the real tragedy of indifference: it is not just an individual failure - it is the result of a system that no longer protects what should be sacred to it.

5. The path to authenticity - between self-knowledge and structural criticism

Overcoming the gap between aspiration and reality does not begin with change on the outside - but with a process of self-recognition. If you want to preserve humanity, you have to allow yourself to recognise where it is lacking. Those who want to revitalise it must have the courage to admit their own wounds. And those who want to institutionalise it must be prepared to question the structures that hinder it.

This reconnection to the ethical is not a moral appeal - it is an existential movement. It begins in a moment of stillness: in the recognition of one's own ambivalence, one's own exhaustion, one's own loss. It grows in encounters with others who feel the same. And it finds its expression in the shaping of practice - where closeness becomes possible again, where questions are allowed again, where people no longer have to disappear.

Humanity is not saved by programmes, but by attitudes. It is not created through obligation, but through permission. It grows where people recognise themselves and each other as human beings again - in doubt, in courage, in limitation. And this is precisely where its power lies: it is not a state - it is a decision. Again and again. Every day. In the middle of the system.

6. Maturing humanity- a path through ambivalence

The experience of the discrepancy between what should be and what is is one of the most profound psychological stresses in everyday medical work. It confronts helpers not only with external barriers - such as time pressure, overload or structural indifference - but above all with themselves:

with their own ideals, hopes and self-images. When these become internally fragile, two typical reaction patterns emerge: retreating into cynicism or fleeing into exhaustion. Both reactions provide short-term protection - but in the long term they close off the path to genuine human presence.

The way out of this inner impasse does not lie in radically turning away from the ideal, but in maturing. Mature humanity recognises that it is not always completely possible. It accepts the tensions, the limitations, the contradictions - but it does not renounce the ethos of care. It knows that you cannot do justice to everyone, that you make mistakes, that you become numb - and yet it remains connected to the inner intention of being human.

This attitude is not a compromise, but a conscious approach to ambivalence. It consists of understanding the ideal not as an expectation, but as an orientation. Not as a demand that must be fulfilled - but as a reminder of why you have chosen this profession. This form of humanity does not remain pure, intact or always available - but it remains alive. It becomes resistant to coldness because it has learnt to live with its own vulnerability.

Mature humanity is revealed in small gestures that arise from inner clarity: in an apologetic look after a tone that was too harsh. In the decision to listen to a patient after all - despite time pressure. In the willingness to remain honest even when it is uncomfortable. In the ability not to play at compassion, but to retrieve it - from the depths of one's own conscience, which has not been dulled by experience, but sharpened.

This attitude cannot be prescribed - but it can grow. It arises when people do not remain alone in their inner ambivalence. When they are allowed to talk about what is missing - without guilt, without shame. When they are recognised for staying - even when it gets difficult. When they experience that there are spaces in which humanity is not only desired, but supported. In such spaces, the contradiction between aspiration and reality does not become a rupture - but a process: honest, open, vulnerable - but connected.

And therein lies the promise of mature humanity: that it is not idealistic, but realistic. Not heroic, but humble. Not tireless, but steadfast. It doesn't need glamour - but a counterpart. Not perfection - but remembrance. And no applause - but a culture in which humanity is not taken for granted, but remains possible. Always anew.

Chapter 20: What remains- The decision for humanity as daily practice

1. The decision as a daily act of resistance

In the medical context, humanity is not a state that can be achieved once and then possessed. It is a process that must constantly prove itself anew under the conditions of routine, time pressure, functional compression and psychological stress. In this respect, humanity is a decision - but not in the sense of a dramatic decision, but as a quiet, everyday act of resistance. Resistance not against people, but against the mechanical. Against slipping into distance. Against the alienation of one's own actions.

This decision is not heroic. It usually happens unnoticed - and often precisely when it has no immediate effect. The empathetic look that the patient is unable to return. The honest word to a colleague that remains unspoken. The moment of pause before the next bed is called. These acts do not immediately change the structure - but they prevent the structure from taking over the inside. They keep the self in touch with what it once wanted.

Its power lies in this repetition: those who decide again and again not to petrify, not to become cynical, not to be indifferent, quietly renew the substance of their profession. They don't become better - but more sincere. Not unassailable - but awake. And this is precisely the ethos that does not radiate outwards, but carries inwards.

2. Unfinished ethics- humanity as an imposition

Those who choose humanity also choose an imposition: to endure tensions, to bear their own limitations, to recognise the imperfection of the system - and their own role in it. It is a mistake to believe that you can live humanity without being hurt. Those who remain open are touched. Those who are touched are hit. And those who are hit are vulnerable.

This imposition is not a weakness - it is a condition. Because only those who expose themselves to this touchability remain in relationship. Only those who don't reject everything can still see. The danger lies not in pain - but in dullness. In the exhaustion that disguises itself with functioning. In the tiredness that becomes an attitude. Humanity does not begin where everything is easy - but where you still don't stop feeling.

In this sense, humanity is never complete. It is an open process. An ethic that can always be interrupted, jeopardised, forgotten - and yet is capable of starting anew. Those who live this ethic do not expect perfection - but presence. Not control - but presence. And it is precisely in this imperfection that its dignity lies.

3. Self-care as a prerequisite for ethical presence

Humanity as a daily practice is only possible if it is not based on self-exploitation. If you want to see others, you must not overlook yourself. Those who care for others must not neglect themselves. Self-care is not a selfish deviation - it is an ethical necessity. Because the self that sacrifices itself eventually loses its voice. And without a voice, there is no testimony. Without testimony, no relationship. Without relationship, no humanity.

Self-care does not mean wellness - it means being aware of your own limits. It means being able to say no. Accepting help. Taking tiredness seriously. Not out of withdrawal, but out of responsibility. A person who is exhausted can no longer empathise. A voice that is constantly overheard falls silent. The decision in favour of humanity is therefore also a decision against self-forgetfulness.

This realisation is central - and yet rarely part of professional identity. Because those who feel called want to give. But if you don't receive, you lose. Those who are not held fall apart. Those who are only allowed to be strong become deaf to their own. That is why the institution is obliged to protect those who protect. Spaces of relief, clarification and recognition are not a bonus - they are the condition for humanity to survive.

4. The silent responsibility of the institution

Humanity is often individualised - as an attitude, a question of character, a virtue. But it is also a systemic issue. No one can act humanly in the long term in an environment that dehumanises them. Structures that leave no room for relationships, that prohibit conversation, that mistrust closeness, prevent ethics - not through commandment, but through organisation. This is why the institution bears responsibility - not just for processes, but for the atmosphere.

A clinic that wants humanity must create conditions in which it is possible. This begins with time windows in which listening can take place. It continues in the culture of interaction - with hierarchy, with mistakes, with grief. And it is reflected in the language: Do we talk about patients or with them? Do we talk about colleagues - or with them? Is closeness encouraged or treated as a risk?

Institutions that do not ask these questions will not recognise indifference - because they do not develop a sense for it. However, institutions that make such questions part of their culture enable change - not abruptly, but sustainably. They not only protect patients - but also those who are there for them. And in doing so, they make a contribution that goes beyond management: they preserve humanity as a collective value.

5. What remains- in the depths

At the end of the reflection, there is no simple formula. No guarantee. No final answer. What remains is a movement - an inner questioning that does not stop. A quiet realisation that humanity must be reborn again and again - in conversation, in the gaze, in the decision not to be indifferent. And that it dies when no one asks any more questions.

What remains is perhaps this: that it is not strength not to feel. No wisdom not to doubt. No efficiency not to touch. What remains is the human being - not as an ideal image, but as a being that does not lose itself because it remembers. That does not close itself off because it is wounded. That does not stop because it is tired. Instead, it remains - in all its fragility, but with an open heart.

And that is exactly what counts: not heroism, but loyalty. Not the smooth, but the true. Not the great, but the next. The decision in favour of humanity is a silent decision. But it is the most important one you can make every day.

Preserving humanity- despite everything

This book is not an indictment. It is an attempt to make something visible that too often remains invisible: the quiet, often unnoticed transformation of a healing profession into a functioning system. The daily shift from compassion to mechanics. The transformation of relationship into routine. The replacement of sensing with doing. Indifference is not the enemy from without - it is a shadow that grows from within when conditions that enable humanity are lacking.

Indifference does not kill in a single moment. It kills slowly, insidiously, over years: the joy of encounter, the power of meaning, the alertness for the special. It not only kills compassion for others - it also undermines compassion for oneself. In the end, what remains is a person who no longer knows why they once started out.

And yet this book is not a gloomy account. It is also a testimony to hope: that humanity has not disappeared - it is just hidden. That it is not lost - but wounded. That it is not impossible - but challenging. That it doesn't have to be perfect - but tangible. Again and again.

Humanity is not a constant, but a movement. It is not an attitude, but a daily endeavour. Not a possession, but a relationship to oneself, to others and to the world that needs to be constantly cultivated. If you want to live it, you don't need ideals, you need connection. Not explanations, but presence. Not superiority, but honesty.

The path back to humanity does not lead via moral superiority. It leads through vulnerability. Through the ability to say: I'm tired. I'm not always there. I want more. And by deciding not to give up anyway. Humanity is when someone stays - even when it's hard. When someone listens - even when everything is talking. When someone acts - not out of duty, but out of solidarity.

The medicine of the future will not be measured by how many devices it masters, how many standards it adheres to, how many processes it optimises. It will be measured by how many people it allows to remain human. And that starts with each individual. Every day. Quietly.

Outlook: A medicine that heals - not just the body

What follows from the above? Certainly not that everything needs to be rethought. Nor that humanity can be secured through reforms alone. But rather this: that it is time to broaden our view. Humanity must no longer be seen as a mere ideal - it must be understood as a structural necessity.

This means that we don't need more guiding principles, but spaces. Spaces in which we can speak, listen, doubt and ask questions. Spaces in which the uncertain has a place. Where leadership also means protecting. Where learning also means feeling. Where work is not just a process, but an encounter.

A new form of training is needed: one that understands emotional self-awareness not as a disorder, but as a resource. One that teaches ethical reflection not as a side issue, but as the centrepiece of practice. One in which young people do not unlearn what once led them to the profession.

We need a new culture of collegiality: open, approachable, responsible. A culture in which people don't have to prove themselves, but are allowed to show themselves. In which people don't withdraw when they have doubts, but come closer. In which the shared silence about what is missing is replaced by shared dialogue about what is possible.

And we need a policy that recognises that a healthcare system is only sustainable if it allows the people who work in it to remain fully human. Not as an ideal, but as a basic condition for quality, safety and the future.

The return to humanity is not a romantic idea. It is a concrete necessity. It does not begin with a major reform - but with a small decision. Now. In this moment. In the next encounter.

Because what heals was never just technology. But always: the other person.